SO-BTB-800

Secondary Data Sources for Public Health
A Practical Guide

Secondary data play an increasingly important role in epidemiology and public health research and practice; examples of secondary data sources include national surveys such as the BRFSS and NHIS, claims data for the Medicare and Medicaid systems, and public vital statistics records. Although a wealth of secondary data is available, it is not always easy to locate and access appropriate data to address a research or policy question.

This practical guide circumvents these difficulties by providing an introduction to secondary data and issues specific to its management and analysis, followed by an enumeration of major sources of secondary data in the United States. Entries for each data source include the principal focus of the data, years for which it is available, history and methodology of the data collection process, and information about how to access the data and supporting materials, including relevant details about file structure and format.

Sarah Boslaugh received her PhD from the City University of New York and her MPH from Saint Louis University. She is currently a Performance Research Analyst for BJC Healthcare in Saint Louis and an Adjunct Professor at the Washington University School of Medicine. She previously worked as a biostatistician and methodologist at Montefiore Medical Center in New York City, Saint Louis University School of Public Health, and the Washington University School of Medicine in Saint Louis. She has also written *An Intermediate Guide to SPSS Programming: Using Syntax for Data Management* (2004) and is Editor-in-Chief of the *Encyclopedia of Epidemiology* (2007).

Practical Guides to Biostatistics and Epidemiology

Series advisors
Susan Ellenberg, *University of Pennsylvania School of Medicine*
Robert C. Elston, *Case Western Reserve University School of Medicine*
Brian Everitt, *Institute for Psychiatry, King's College London*
Frank Harrell, *Vanderbilt University Medical Center*
Jos W. R. Twisk, *Vrije Universiteit Medical Centre, Amsterdam*

This is a series of short and practical but authoritative books for biomedical researchers, clinical investigators, public health researchers, epidemiologists, and nonacademic and consulting biostatisticians who work with data from biomedical and epidemiological and genetic studies. Some books are explorations of a modern statistical method and its application; others focus on a particular disease or condition and the statistical techniques most commonly used in studying it.

This series is for people who use statistics to answer specific research questions. The books explain the application of techniques, specifically the use of computational tools, and emphasize the interpretation of results, not the underlying mathematical and statistical theory.

Published in the series
Applied Multilevel Analysis, by **Jos W. R. Twisk**

Secondary Data Sources for Public Health

A Practical Guide

Sarah Boslaugh

BJC Healthcare

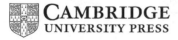

CAMBRIDGE
UNIVERSITY PRESS

CAMBRIDGE UNIVERSITY PRESS
Cambridge, New York, Melbourne, Madrid, Cape Town, Singapore, São Paulo

Cambridge University Press
32 Avenue of the Americas, New York, NY 10013-2473, USA

www.cambridge.org
Information on this title: www.cambridge.org/9780521870016

First published 2007

Printed in the United States of America

A catalog record for this publication is available from the British Library.

Library of Congress Cataloging in Publication Data

Boslaugh, Sarah.
Secondary data sources for public health : a practical guide / Sarah Boslaugh.
   p. ; cm. – (Practical guides to biostatistics and epidemiology)
Includes bibliographical references and index.
ISBN-13: 978-0-521-87001-6 (hardback)
ISBN-10: 0-521-87001-1 (hardback)
ISBN-13: 978-0-521-69023-2 (pbk.)
ISBN-10: 0-521-69023-4 (pbk.)
1. Public health – Research – Statistical methods.   2. Epidemiology – Research –
Statistical methods.   I. Title.   II. Series.
[DNLM: 1. Data Collection – United States.   2. Epidemiology – United States.
3. Public Health – United States. WA 950 B743s   2007]
RA409.B66   2007
362.1072′7–dc22   2006034301

ISBN   978-0-521-87001-6 hardback
ISBN   978-0-521-69023-2 paperback

Contents

Preface

Secondary data analysis – meaning, in the broadest sense, analysis of data collected by someone else – plays a vital role in modern epidemiology and public health research and practice. This is partly because of the emphasis on population-based studies that is common to both fields. For instance, few individual researchers could hope to collect data sufficient to evaluate changes in the health status or health behaviors on a national scale. Fortunately, a wealth of data on health and related subjects, collected on a broad scale and over many years, is available for public use. However, locating secondary data appropriate to address a particular research question is not always easy, partly because an abundance of data is available and also because those data were collected by many different entities and are stored in many different locations. My primary purpose in writing *Secondary Data Sources for Public Health* is to facilitate use of those data sets in epidemiologic and public health research.

Chapter 1 introduces the topic of secondary data analysis, discusses some of its advantages and disadvantages, describes a general process for locating appropriate data to address a research question, and suggests some types of information that the researcher should try to acquire about any secondary data set being considered for analysis. Chapters 2 through 7 discuss the major secondary data sets and data archives available for studying health issues in the United States. These chapters are organized thematically, so Chapter 2 discusses health service utilization data; Chapter 3, health behaviors and risk factors data; Chapter 4, data sets dealing with multiple health topics; Chapter 5, fertility and mortality data; Chapter 6, Medicare and Medicaid data; and Chapter 7, other sources of data. The bibliography is organized by chapter and lists a number of works, primarily theoretical and methodologic, relating to secondary data analysis and the data sets discussed. Appendix I lists the acronyms used in this volume, with the full name of the entity referred to and, if applicable, places the acronym in context. For instance, a term may be used primarily in conjunction with a particular data set, or a data set may be part of a larger project. Appendix II summarizes the data sets discussed in this volume, including the years for which data are available. Appendix III discusses data import and transfer.

Acknowledgments

This book would not have been written without the assistance and support of many individuals. In particular, I thank Elena Andresen for introducing me to secondary data analysis when I was a student at the Saint Louis University School of Public Health and for her steadfast belief in my abilities; Rand Ross at Washington University for helping me preserve my sanity; Neil Salkind, my agent at Studio B, for his unflagging support; Lauren Cowles, my editor at Cambridge University Press, for her patience and encouragement; and my husband, Dan Peck, for being there through it all.

An Introduction to Secondary Data Analysis

What Are Secondary Data?

In the fields of epidemiology and public health, the distinction between *primary* and *secondary* data depends on the relationship between the person or research team who collected a data set and the person who is analyzing it. This is an important concept because the same data set could be primary data in one analysis and secondary data in another. If the data set in question was collected by the researcher (or a team of which the researcher is a part) for the specific purpose or analysis under consideration, it is *primary data*. If it was collected by someone else for some other purpose, it is *secondary data*. Of course, there will always be cases in which this distinction is less clear, but it may be useful to conceptualize primary and secondary data by considering two extreme cases. In the first, which is an example of *primary data*, a research team conceives of and develops a research project, collects data designed to address specific questions posed by the project, and performs and publishes their own analyses of the data they have collected. In this case, the people involved in analyzing the data have some involvement in, or at least familiarity with, the research design and data collection process, and the data were collected to answer the questions examined in the analysis. In the second case, which is an example of *secondary data*, a researcher poses questions that are addressed through analysis of data from the Behavioral Risk Factor Surveillance System (BRFSS), a data set collected annually in the United States through cooperation of the Centers for Disease Control and Prevention and state health departments. In this case, the person performing the analysis did not participate in either the research design or data collection process, and the data were not collected to answer specific research questions.

As an example of the same data set serving as both primary and secondary data, consider the increasingly common practice of one researcher performing an analysis of data collected by a research team with whom he or she has no connection. This type of analysis is facilitated by the ease of sharing data stored electronically and the concomitant creation of electronic data archives that allow access to secondary users; some of these archives are discussed in Chapter 7. Such analyses may serve a variety of purposes, such as addressing questions not considered in the original analysis or examining how a different analytic approach might change the conclusions reached from the first analysis. In either case, the same data set serves as *primary data* for the original research team and *secondary data* for the researcher performing the later analysis.

This book deals primarily with secondary data in the sense of data sets that can be obtained and analyzed in detail by the individual researcher. There is another type of secondary data, again not mutually exclusive with the first, meaning statistical information about some geographic region or other entity. This type of information is often useful to researchers: when you place your research project in context by describing the racial makeup or median house value in the metropolitan area where you conduct your research, the data used to compute those statistics were probably secondary data. Often these statistics are computed on data collected by the federal government, and Chapter 7 discusses several websites that were created specifically to permit easy access to these types of statistics. In addition, many of the data sets described in this book are accessible through an online interface that allows the quick computation of basic statistics, without requiring the user to download data and use a statistical program to analyze it. The availability of such interfaces has been noted in the sections pertaining to each data set.

Most of the data sets discussed in this volume contain either data collected through surveys or censuses, such as the National Health Interview Survey and the U.S. Census, or administrative records such as the medical claims records submitted to the Medicare system. There are other types of secondary data, including diaries, videorecordings, and transcripts of interviews and focus groups: some of these are included in sources discussed in Chapter 7. Data such as interview transcripts are often analyzed using qualitative data methods rather than the quantitative techniques appropriate for most of the data sets discussed in this volume. Secondary analysis of qualitative data is a topic unto itself and is not discussed in this volume. The interested reader is referred to references such as James and Sorenson (2000) and Heaton (2004).

Advantages and Disadvantages of Secondary Data Analysis

The choice of primary or secondary data need not be an either/or question. Most researchers in epidemiology and public health will work with both types of data in the course of their careers, and many research projects incorporate both types of data. A more useful approach to this question is to focus on selecting data that are appropriate to the research question being studied and the resources available to the researcher; the latter include time, money, and personal expertise. In this spirit, we offer a summary of the major advantages and disadvantages of working with secondary, as opposed to primary, data.

The first major advantage of working with secondary data is economy: because someone else has already collected the data, the researcher does not have to devote resources to this phase of research. Even if the secondary data set must be purchased, the cost is almost certainly lower than the expense of salaries, transportation, and so forth that would be required to collect and process a similar data set from scratch. There is also a savings of time. Because the data are already collected, and frequently also cleaned and stored in electronic format, the researcher can spend the bulk of his or her time analyzing the data. There is also the influence of preference: secondary data analysis is an ideal focus for researchers who prefer to spend their working hours thinking of and testing hypotheses using existing data sets, rather than writing grants to finance the data collection process and supervising student interviewers and data entry clerks.

The second major advantage of using secondary data is the breadth of data available. Few individual researchers would have the resources to collect data from a representative sample of adults in every state in the

United States, let alone repeat this data collection process every year, but the federal government conducts numerous surveys on that scale. Data collected on a national basis are particularly important in epidemiology and public health, fields that focus primarily on the health of populations rather than of individuals. In addition, some of the data sets discussed in Chapters 2 through 7 collect data using a longitudinal design, and others are designed so certain questions are included annually or at regular intervals, allowing researchers to examine the changes in health status and health behaviors in the population over time.

The third advantage in using secondary data is that often the data collection process is informed by expertise and professionalism that may not available to smaller research projects. For instance, many of the federal health surveys discussed in this volume use a complex sample design and system of weighting that allows the researcher to compute population-based estimates of health conditions and behaviors. Although a local data collection project could conceivably use similar techniques, more often a convenience sample, whose generalizability is questionable, is used instead. To take another example, data collection for many federal data sets is often performed by staff members who specialize in that task and who may have years of experience working on a particular survey. This is in contrast to many smaller research projects, in which data are collected by students working at a part-time, temporary job.

One major disadvantage to using secondary data is inherent in its nature: because the data were not collected to answer your specific research questions, particular information that you would like to have may not have been collected. Or it may not have been collected in the geographic region you want to study, in the years you would have chosen, or on the specific population that is the focus of your interest. In any case, you can only work with the data that exist, not what you wish had been collected. A related problem is that variables may have been defined or categorized differently than you would have chosen: for instance, a data set may have collected age information in categories rather than as a continuous variable, or race may have been defined as only White/Other. A third difficulty is that data may have been collected but are not available to the secondary researcher: for instance, address and phone number information for survey respondents may have been recorded by the original research team but will not be released to secondary researchers for confidentiality reasons. If an analysis incorporating geographic information was planned, such a restriction might make the data set unusable. For these reasons, a secondary data set should be examined carefully to confirm that it includes the necessary data, that the data are defined and coded in a manner that allows for the desired analysis, and that the researcher will be allowed to access the data required.

A second major disadvantage of using secondary data is that because the analyst did not participate in the planning and execution of the data collection process, he or she does not know exactly how it was done. More to the point, the analyst does not know how well it was done and therefore how seriously the data are affected by problems such as low response rate or respondent misunderstanding of specific survey questions. Every data collection effort has its "dirty little secrets" that may not invalidate the data but should be taken into account by the analyst. If the analyst was not present during the data collection process, he or she has to try to find this information through other means. Sometimes it is readily available; for instance, many of the federal data sets have extensive documentation of their data collection procedures, refusal rates, and other technical information available on their websites or in published reports. However, many other secondary data sets are not accompanied by this type of information, and the analyst must learn to "read between the lines" and consider what problems might have been encountered in the data collection process.

Locating Appropriate Secondary Data

There is a vast quantity of secondary data in epidemiology and public health that is available to the individual researcher. However, the sheer quantity of data available, and the fact that the data are collected and archived by many different governmental and private entities, means that the process of locating appropriate secondary data is not always straightforward. In fact, this book was written to ameliorate some of the difficulties involved. There is no single process to be followed in every case, but we offer two examples of the process of locating and analyzing secondary data to address a specific research question or problem.

This section might have been better titled "achieving a fit between your research question and the data you choose to analyze" because it is often an iterative process in which a research question is posed, potential data sets are considered, the question is refined in terms of the data available, other sources of data are considered, the question is refined again, and so on. The most typical way to use secondary data for research is to begin with a research question and seek a data set that will allow analysis of that question. An alternative method is to begin by selecting from among the available secondary data sets, and then formulating a research question that may be answered using the data chosen. Although the first method conforms more to standard beliefs about how research is done, the second approach is particularly useful in classroom instruction, and both methods can produce quality research. If the researcher begins with a question and then seeks out an appropriate data set, the following generalized sequence of procedures may be useful:

1. Define the question you want to study; for instance, "How does the experience of racism affect an individual's health?"
2. Specify the population you want to study. Are you interested in children, adults, or people of all ages? What races or ethnicities do you want to study? Do you want to analyze a national sample or one confined to a smaller area? What is the range of years you would consider (e.g., you may only be interested in data collected over the last 5 years)?
3. Specify what other variables you want to include in your analysis. In this example, you might believe that it was important to have information about the respondents' race, Hispanic ethnicity, age, gender, income, and educational level in order to include those factors in your analysis. If so, you must confirm that the data you desire are contained in the data set that you choose and that they are recorded in a manner that is useful to you. If you are interested in comparing the experiences of Hispanic Blacks and non-Hispanic Blacks, information about Hispanic ethnicity would need to be recorded in the data set independently of information about race.
4. Specify what kind of data is most appropriate for your research question: for instance, can it best be addressed through a national survey, examination of hospital claims records, or transcriptions of

interviews? Also, specify if there are any specific data collection techniques you believe are particularly appropriate or inappropriate for your question. For instance, if you do not believe people would answer questions about racism honestly in a personal interview, you would not consider any data sets collected using that technique. However, if you believe that a telephone survey would be the best way to collect this information, you might begin your search by looking at surveys that used this data collection method.

5. Create a list of data sets that include information related to your research question and examine them to see if they meet your other requirements (age range included, year of collection, etc.). This is where the interactive process begins because you may have to revise either your question or your data requirements, depending on the data that are available to you.

6. Once you have chosen your data set, examine the variables you intend to use for the analysis of problems such as missing data or out-of-range values. Also, read whatever information you can find about the data collection process, data cleaning procedures, and so on in order to evaluate whether the data quality is sufficient to meet your needs. If so, continue with the analysis; if not, either devise a way to work around it (e.g., by imputing values for the missing data) or choose another data set.

How do you generate the list mentioned in step five? By any means necessary, as the saying goes. Consider the data sets described in this book, search Medline to see what data sets other researchers have used to address your topic, search the web portals listed in Chapter 7, ask other researchers for suggestions, query relevant email lists, and so forth.

If you take the approach of beginning with a data set and crafting a research question that can be addressed using it, the process is similar, but the order of events is different. In this case, you would begin by looking at the variables contained in the data set and considering how you might combine them to create an interesting question. The process can begin with a germ of an idea, which may reflect your personal interests or a question that has arisen in your work. For instance, you might be interested in how disability affects the amount of physical activity in which a person engages. You then need to operationalize this question so it may be tested using the variables available in the data set: how will you define disability, and how will you define physical activity? At this point, a Medline search for related articles would be in order, to see how others have addressed similar questions and whether they have done so with the data set you will be using. This step will help keep you from reinventing the wheel and will place your research in context.

Alternatively, you can begin by simply looking at the variables included in the data set to see which of them interest you. For instance, if you were planning to work with the BRFSS data from 2005, you might notice that eleven states included questions on weight control procedures. You would then look at the actual questions asked and confirm that the data were actually available. Information to answer both questions can be found on the BRFSS website (http://www.cdc.gov/brfss). This process should help you refine your focus so you can craft a research question that can be answered using BRFSS 2005 data and that would add to our understanding of public health. Because the BRFSS includes racial and ethnic data, you might decide to look at racial and ethnic differences in weight control practices. Or, taking advantage of the fact that BRFSS data are identified by state of residence, you could plan to conduct a comparison of weight control practices in different states. You could also plan a multilevel analysis that combined information about state-level characteristics from the U.S. Census (e.g., racial makeup or poverty level) with the individual-level data available in the BRFSS. When you have selected the variables you will include in your analysis, confirm that they are coded (or can be recoded by you) in a manner that will support your intended analysis and that there are no major data quality issues such as large quantities of missing data.

Questions to Ask About Any Secondary Data Set

Once you have located a secondary data set that you think is appropriate for your analysis, you need to learn as much as you can about why and how it was collected. In particular, you will want to answer the following three questions:

1. What was the original purpose for which the data were collected?
2. What kind of data is it, and when and how were the data collected?
3. What cleaning and/or recoding procedures have been applied to the data?

Sources for this information include the website of the agency or other entity responsible for collecting and/or making the data available, published reports, research articles based on the data, and personal communications with relevant individuals. For instance, many of the federal agency websites include one or more contact people who are available to answer questions about the data collected by that agency, and a Medline search will often produce citations to reports and articles discussing the procedures used to collect particular data sets.

The question of determining the original purpose of the project that produced the data is important because its influence may be present in other characteristics of the data, from the population targeted to the specific wording of questions included in a survey. Because you were not involved in planning phases for the project whose data you will analyze, you need this information in order to place the data in context. To take an extreme case, you would certainly want to know if a research project on the health effects of smoking was sponsored by a tobacco company or by a nonprofit dedicated to smoking prevention. You would also like to know if there was any particular philosophy or model of health behavior that shaped the project: for instance, was a smoking cessation program structured using the Transtheoretical Model? Knowledge of the core philosophical beliefs behind a research project can illuminate the reasons for many choices made in the planning and execution of the research and will be reflected in the end product, the data you are proposing to analyze.

It is almost impossible to know too much about the data collection process because it can influence the quality of the data in many ways, some of them not obvious. To start with, you need to know when the data were collected. A data set released in 2004 may have been collected in the first 3 months of 2004 or over a 4-year period from 2000 to 2003. Second, you want to know the process by which the data were collected: was it via telephone interviews, in-person interviews, abstraction of hospital records, or some other technique? Third, you want to know the details of the data collection process. Questions in this regard include who actually did the data collection, how extensive was their training, and how carefully were they supervised. If the data were collected through chart review, what specific instructions were given to the reviewers? If the data were collected through a survey, what was the response rate? How many efforts were made to collect data from nonresponders? If data were collected through a telephone survey, how were numbers selected? Was there any attempt to correct for the bias introduced because households without a telephone are not a random sample of all households? The issues of survey data quality are the same whether the data set is primary or secondary. For a thorough discussion of these issues, consult a reference such as de Vaus (2002) or Bulmer, Sturgis, and Allum (2006).

The third major question in working with any secondary data set is what was done to the data after they were collected. For instance, almost all data sets include some missing data. Were these data left as missing, or were values imputed, and if so, how was the imputation done? Was any data cleaning done to remove out-of-range values, and were those cases assigned missing values or was some other procedure followed? Were certain combinations of answers considered invalid, and if so, how were they treated? A famous example of this last type of procedure was the decision in the 1990 U.S. Census to recode to the opposite gender one member of a same-gender couple who declared themselves to be married. If any recoding has been done, is it possible to restore the original values? You also need to find out if data can be weighted, and if so, for what aggregations the weighting allows the production of accurate estimates (e.g., at the national level alone or at both the national and the state levels).

Considerations Relating to Causal Inference

Causality and causal inference are complex topics that can be touched on only briefly here. Issues surrounding causal inference are discussed in greater detail by Rothman and Greenland (1998) and Phillips and Goodman (2006). One of the first rules taught in a basic statistics course is "association does not prove causation," or because A is correlated with B does not mean that A causes B. In the absence of any further information, it is equally plausible that B causes A or that their relationship is caused by a third variable, C, which is related to both A and B but was not included in the analysis. This problem is particularly relevant when analyzing cross-sectional data (i.e., data that are collected at a single point in time). Although the problems surrounding causation exist with both primary and secondary data, because many secondary data sets are cross-sectional, they are particularly relevant for people who work primarily with secondary data.

One way to establish chronology is to use data collected from the same people at several points in time. If A was collected in 1998 and B was collected in 2000, A may have caused B, but B did not cause A. This requires data collected from the same individuals at two or more time points and requires that those individuals can be identified at each time point (not necessarily by name but by some variable that allows the data collected from each person to be identified). This technique may be applied to data such as that collected by the *Medical Expenditures Panel Study*, which collects data about all members of a sampled household or family for 2 years, and in which data for each individual is identified so data from the 2 years may be linked. A second method of establishing chronology is sometimes possible, even for data collected at a single point in time, by considering the time period to which the data refers, rather than when it was collected. For instance, birth certificate data are usually considered cross-sectional because they are collected at one point in time, but some of the data, such as the mother's prenatal care, refer to events that by definition took place before other events, such as the birth. Note that establishing temporal sequence and association does not in and of itself establish causality: such questions can become quite complex and are discussed in detail in Pearl (2000).

2

Health Services Utilization Data

This chapter discusses twelve sources of data about health services utilization at the state, regional, or national level in the United States. The title *National Health Care Survey* (NHCS) actually refers to eight surveys conducted under the auspices of the National Center for Health Statistics (NCHS): the *National Ambulatory Medical Care Survey* (NAMCS), the *National Hospital Ambulatory Medical Care Survey* (NHAMCS), the *National Hospital Discharge Survey* (NHDS), the *National Nursing Home Survey* (NNHS), the *National Health Provider Inventory* (NHPI), the *National Survey of Ambulatory Surgery* (NSAS), the *National Home and Hospice Care Survey* (NHHCS), and the *National Employer Health Insurance Survey* (NEHIS). Three other surveys are also discussed. The *Healthcare Cost and Utilization Project* (HCUP) is a family of databases created from discharge records from community hospitals and ambulatory surgery sites. The *Medical Expenditures Panel Survey* (MEPS) collects data on health care utilization and costs and insurance coverage, and uses an overlapping panel design for the household portion of the survey so data on each participating household are available for 2 full years. The *National Immunization Survey* (NIS) collects data on immunization rates for children ages 19 to 35 months, whenever possible, from both the child's parent or other adult household member and their vaccination provider(s). The *Surveillance Epidemiology and End Results* (SEER) program collects information on cancer incidence, treatment, and survival from a number of population-based cancer registries in the United States, including demographic information about individual patients.

The National Ambulatory Medical Care Survey

The NAMCS is based on a sample of visits to office-based physicians primarily involved in direct patient care. The survey collects data about patients, their symptoms, physician's diagnoses, and medications, using a form filled out by the participating physician. The NAMCS was conducted annually from 1973 to 1981, next in 1985, and annually since 1989.

Focus

The NAMCS collects information about physician office visits, including characteristics of patients seeking treatment, conditions treated, diagnostic and therapeutic services supplied, and medications prescribed or recommended. Because the NAMCS is based on a sample of physician visits rather than a population sample, it cannot be used to estimate the frequency of a particular disease or condition in the U.S. population. However, NAMCS data are used to calculate statistics such as the most common diagnoses, the most common physician services provided, and the number and percent of mentions of particular drugs or classes of drugs, such as antidepressants per 100 physician visits.

Data Collection

NAMCS data are collected from physicians, who fill out a Patient Record form for each of a systematic random sample of their office visits during a randomly assigned 1-week period. Data collection for the NAMCS is overseen by staff from the U.S. Bureau of the Census. Prior to the sampling week, a Census field representative visits the physician to provide him or her with survey materials and instructions on how to complete the forms. Although the information collected has varied somewhat over the years, much of it has remained constant, facilitating the combination or comparison of information collected by the NAMCS in different years.

The NAMCS uses a three-stage probability design:

1. Large geographic areas or primary sampling units (PSUs)
2. Physician practices within PSUs
3. Patient visits within physician practices

Only certain types of physician practices are eligible to be selected in the second stage: the physicians must be nonfederally employed and not working in the specialties of anesthesiology, pathology, or radiology. The third stage of sampling has two parts: the physician practice sample is divided into fifty-two random subsamples, and each subsample is assigned to 1 of 52 weeks in the year. Then, a random sample of visits (from 20 to 100 percent) based on the size of the practice is designated for each physician for that week, so each physician will complete approximately thirty Patient Record forms.

The 2006 Patient Record form collects data in thirteen categories: patient information, including date of birth, gender, race, tobacco use, and expected source of payment; whether the visit was related to an injury, poisoning, or adverse effect of health care; patient's complaint (i.e., the patient's description of his or her reason for visit); continuity of care; physician's diagnosis; height, weight, temperature, and blood pressure; diagnostic and screening services ordered or provided; health education ordered or provided; nonmedication treatment such as physical therapy or psychotherapy ordered or provided; medications and immunizations ordered, supplied, administered, or continued; type of provider seen (physician, nurse, etc.); visit disposition (e.g., return visit, admit to hospital); and time spent with provider. Most data are supplied by the physician checking one or more boxes; however, reason for visit, diagnosis, and medications and immunizations are all free-text fields that are later coded by survey staff. Some fields are coded using standard references such as the *Ninth Revision of the International Classification of Diseases, Clinical Modification* (ICD-9_CM) used to code diagnoses since 1979. Others, such as patient complaint, are coded using systems developed by the NCHS. Drugs mentioned, including both prescription and over-the-counter medications are also coded using an NCHS classification system, and are further categorized by therapeutic class and by their generic name. Information about drug mentions was kept in a separate data file for the years 1973 to 1991. With 1991 data, it became possible to link drug information to visit information, and since 1992, data about drug mentions have been included in the same data file as the patient visit information.

NAMCS data are designed to provide national estimates of ambulatory case use rather than accurate estimates of disease rates at the state or local level. To maintain confidentiality, public-use NAMCS data files are stripped of geographic identifying information beyond the four Census geographic regions (Northeast, Midwest, South, or West) and about whether the visit took place in a metropolitan statistical area.

Accessing Data and Ancillary Materials

Public-use NAMCS data files and ancillary materials are available for download from the NCHS website (http://www.cdc.gov/nchs/about/major/ahcd/ahcd1.htm). They are also available from the Interuniversity Consortium for Political and Social Research (ICPSR) website (http://webapp.icpsr.umich.edu/cocoon/ICPSR-SERIES/00037.xml). NAMCS data may also be requested on CD-ROM from the NCHS (subject to availability) or purchased from the Government Printing Office (GPO) (http://bookstore.gpo.gov/). Ancillary materials available from the NCHS website include survey instruments; SAS, SPSS, and Stata syntax files; documentation regarding the survey process and data sets; a number of educational presentations on topics such as "Using NAMCS Data for Injury Analysis"; and a bibliography of publications using NAMCS data.

Under certain circumstances, researchers may be granted access to NAMCS data files that include more identifying information (i.e., to files containing data that are masked in the publicly available data sets because of confidentiality concerns). Researchers must apply through the Research Data Center (RDC) at NCHS for access to these files, by submitting a proposal detailing why they need access to the more specific data files. More information about this process is available from the Centers for Disease Control and Prevention (CDC) website (http://www.cdc.gov/nchs/data/ahcd/NAMCSandNHAMCSDataAvailable.pdf).Types of data on the files available through the RDC include characteristics of physician practices such as size and sources of revenue, physician demographic characteristics, state and county Federal Information Processing Standards (FIPS) codes, patient ZIP code (beginning in 2005), and characteristics of the patient's ZIP code as drawn from U.S. Census data.

The National Hospital Ambulatory Medical Care Survey

The NHAMCS is a national survey based on a sample of visits to hospital outpatient department (OPDs) and emergency departments (EDs). The NHAMCS has been conducted annually since 1992, and collects patient demographic information, triage information, patient's complaint, and physician's diagnosis, as well as services, procedures, and medications and immunizations provided.

Focus

In many ways, the NHAMCS can be considered as an extension of or supplement to the NAMCS. In fact, NHAMCS data collection began in 1992, after health researchers realized that patient visits to hospital OPDs and EDs, which are excluded from the NAMCS, were supplying an ever greater proportion of the nation's ambulatory care. The NHAMCS is intended to provide nationally accurate estimates of ambulatory visits to hospital OPDs and EDs.

Data Collection

NHAMCS data are collected on Patient Record forms filled out by hospital staff for a random sample of patient visits during a randomly assigned 4-week reporting period. As with the NAMCS, the field data collection is overseen by employees of the U.S. Bureau of the Census. The NHAMCS uses a four-stage probability design:

1. Large geographic areas or PSUs
2. Hospitals within PSUs
3. Clinics within hospitals
4. Patient visits with clinics

Federal, military, and Veterans Administration hospitals are excluded from the NHAMCS, as are hospital units of institutions (e.g., prisons) and hospitals with fewer than six staffed patient beds. A fixed panel of 600 hospitals was selected at random for the NHAMCS in 1991. This panel was updated in 2001 to include hospitals that had opened or changed their eligibility status since 1991. The hospital sample was divided into sixteen subsets, and each was assigned one of sixteen 4-week reporting periods, beginning on December 2, 1991. The reporting periods rotate across each reporting year so each hospital is included approximately once every 15 months. Within a 4-week period, patient visits are systematically selected (every nth visit after a random starting point), based on expected patient volume, with the goal of having each hospital complete 100 Patient Record forms for visits to the ED and 200 for the OPD.

The ED and OPD Patient Record forms are similar but not identical, both to each other and to the NAMCS Patient Record. The 2005 NHAMCS ED Patient Record collects data in twelve categories: patient information, including date of birth, gender, race, mode of arrival, and expected source of payment; triage information, including vital signs, level of pain, and immediacy of need for care; previous hospital or ED care; patient's complaint; if visit was related to an injury, poisoning, or adverse effect of health care; physician's diagnosis; diagnostic or screening services provided; procedures performed; medications and immunizations given or prescribed; providers seen; visit disposition; and hospital admission. The 2005 OPD Patient Record omits questions about mode of arrival and hospital admission, and includes a section on both health education and nonmedication treatment ordered or provided. Coding of data collected in the free response fields (i.e., patient's complaint, physician diagnosis, and medication and immunizations) is performed as described in the section on the NAMCS.

Accessing Data and Ancillary Materials

Public-use data files and ancillary materials are available for download from the NCHS website (see the previous section on the NAMCS for details).

The National Hospital Discharge Survey

The NHDS collects data from a national sample of records of patients discharged from short-stay, nonfederal hospitals. The NHDS has been conducted annually since 1965, and about 270,000 records are sampled in a given year, from a national sample of about 500 hospitals. Data collected include patient demographics, source of payment, discharge status, length of stay, diagnoses, and procedures performed.

Focus

The NHDS was the first survey of medical care delivery conducted by the NCHS, and remains the principal source of national data about discharges from short-stay, nonfederal hospitals in the fifty states and the District of Columbia. As such, it is used to calculate national estimates of hospital use in the United States, including the number and percent of discharges and average length of stay, the average length of stay for particular diagnostic categories, and the number and rate of particular procedures. The NHDS is also used to calculate trends in hospital utilization, with breakdowns by gender and age category.

Data Collection

From 1965 to 1984, NHDS data were drawn from hospital records and entered on an abstract form, either by a hospital employee or by employees of the U.S. Bureau of the Census on behalf of the NCHS. Beginning in 1985, automated data collection was also used, originally for about 17 percent of the sample hospitals. The automated data collection was conducted through NCHS purchase of medical record data in machine-readable form from hospitals, hospital associations, state data systems, or commercial organizations.

The NHDS used a two-stage sampling technique from 1965 to 1987. For those years, a random sample of hospitals was drawn used a sampling frame of all short-stay (average length of stay less than 30 days), nonfederal hospitals in the United States, stratified according to bed size and geographic location. Within selected hospitals, a systematic random sample of discharges was chosen. The sampling ratio for discharges varied inversely with the probability selection of the hospital so the probability selection for a given discharge was constant across all sizes of hospitals.

In 1988, the sampling procedure was redesigned, and a three-stage sample process was implemented that was linked with the design of the *National Health Interview Survey* (NHIS) to reduce field costs. The sampling stages are

1. Large geographic PSUs, which are a subsample of the PSUs chosen for the NHIS
2. Hospitals within PSUs
3. Patient records within hospitals

Because of the greater efficiency of working with automated data, the target sample size is 250 discharges from hospitals that provide records through manual extraction and 2000 from hospitals that provide automated data.

Data collected for the 2004 NHDS include length of stay; patient demographic information, including age, gender, ethnicity, race, and marital status; type of admission, such as emergency or elective; source of admission, such as physician admission or transfer from the ED; disposition of patient; expected source of payment; physician diagnoses; and surgical and diagnostic procedures performed.

Accessing Data and Ancillary Materials

NHDS data for the years 1996 to 2004 is available for free download from the NCHS FTP server, accessible through the NCHS website at http://www.cdc.gov/nchs/about/major/hdasd/nhds.htm. Each year of data is documented by a detailed report available from the same website. Data for the years 1970 to 1997 is available on CD-ROM and data for the years 1985 to 1994 on diskette for purchase from the National Technical Information Service (NTIS) and/or the GPO. Details are available from the NCHS website (http://www.cdc.gov/nchs/products/elec_prods/subject/nhds.htm).

Other National Health Care Survey Data Sets

The other five parts of the NHCS collect data less frequently, focus on information of a more specialized nature, and are therefore dealt with more briefly in this section.

The *National Nursing Home Survey* (NNHS) was one of the original four elements of the NHCS. It was first conducted in 1973 to 1974, and has since been conducted in the years 1977, 1985, 1995, 1997, 1999, and 2004. A two-stage probability sampling plan is used: selection of nursing homes, and then selection of residents and discharges within nursing homes. Data are collected from staff and administrators, rather than residents, through interviews and self-administered questionnaires. The NNHS collects data on both facilities and residents. Data collected on nursing home facilities include size, ownership, and occupancy rate. Data collected on nursing home residents, both current and discharged, include demographics, health status, and services received. NNHS data in SAS, ASCII, and tab-delimited formats is available for free download for the years 1995, 1997, 1999, and 2004 from the NCHS website (http://www.cdc.gov/nchs/nnhs.htm). Ancillary materials available from the same website include the questionnaires used in those years, SAS and SPSS syntax, and a document describing each year's survey procedures, including sampling techniques and estimation procedures used.

The *National Health Provider Inventory* (NHPI) was also an original component of the NHCS. It is, as the name suggests, an inventory rather than a survey, and provides a comprehensive national listing of health care providers as of 1991, the only year it was conducted. NHPI data were collected via mail questionnaires, and two different forms were used. Nursing homes and board and care homes were sent Facility questionnaires, whereas home health agencies and hospices were sent Agency questionnaires. Both collected similar information, except as noted. Information collected by the NHPI includes location, staff, total number of clients served in 1990, age and gender of residents (Facility questionnaire only), and number of current and discharged clients. The NHPI has served as a sampling frame, as well as a source of data, for other health care provider inventories. NHPI data are available only on tape and must be purchased from the NTIS. Data from the Facility and Agency questionnaires are stored on separate tapes.

The *National Survey of Ambulatory Surgery* (NSAS) was conducted only three times, in 1994, 1995, and 1996. It collects information about ambulatory, as opposed to inpatient, surgery performed in hospitals and freestanding ambulatory surgery centers (FSASCs). Surgery facilities dedicated exclusively to dentistry, podiatry, abortion, pain, or small procedures were excluded, as were facilities that performed less than fifty ambulatory surgery procedures per year. A two-stage sampling probability sampling design was used: hospitals and FSASCs were sampled, and then ambulatory surgery visits were sampled within selected facilities. NSAS data were abstracted from patient medical records and included patient demographic information; expected source of payment; time spent in different phases of care; type of anesthesia used; final diagnoses; and surgical and diagnostic procedures performed. NSAS data are available for purchase on CD-ROM from the NTIS: each year can be purchased separately or as a set containing data from all 3 years. The 3-year data set is also available for purchase from the GPO. Ancillary technical information about the data are included on the CD-ROMs.

The *National Home and Hospice Care Survey* (NHHCS) was conducted in 1992, 1993, 1994, 1996, 1998, and 2000. Three types of data were collected from administrator and staff interviews: information about institutions, including hospices; information about current residents; and information about discharged residents. Two types of institutions were included in the NNHCS: home health agencies and hospices. *Home health agencies* are defined as those who provide care in an individual's place of residence for the purpose of restoring or maintaining health or minimizing the effects of illness or disability. *Hospices* are defined as those that provide palliative and supportive care services for a dying person and their families, in either the person's home or in a specialized facility. A two-stage probability sampling procedure was used to select first institutions, then current residents and discharges within institutions. Data collected by the NHHCS concerning institutions include ownership, certification, number of patients seen, and number and types of staff members. Data collected about current and discharged patients include demographic characteristics, functional status, health status, payment information, and services used. Data and documentation for the years 1992, 1993, 1994, 1996, and 1998 are available for purchase on CD-ROM from the NTIS.

The *National Employer Health Insurance Survey* (NEHIS) collected data about employer-sponsored health insurance and was conducted only once in 1994. The NEHIS surveyed a probability sample of all employers in the United States, including business establishments (e.g., a single General Motors plant in a specific geographic location), governments, and self-employed individuals. A second stage of sampling was applied to employers who offered a large number of insurance plans to their employees: in this case, up to five plans per employer were selected at random. The NEHIS methodology allows valid estimates to be computed at the level of the individual state and at the national level. Information collected by the NEHIS includes availability of employer-sponsored health insurance, characteristics of plans offered, benefits available, and costs. Because of confidentiality concerns, NEHIS data have not been released to the general public, but researchers may apply for access to them through the RDC of the NCHS.

The Healthcare Cost and Utilization Project

The HCUP is a family of databases developed by the Agency for Healthcare Research and Quality (AHRQ) in cooperation with state governments and private organizations. All HCUP data sets are based on discharge data from community hospitals. Community hospitals are defined as short-term, nonfederal hospitals. Specifically excluded from this definition are military, Veterans Administration, and Indian Health Service hospitals; long-term care hospitals; psychiatric hospitals; chemical dependence treatment units; and hospitals within institutions such as prisons. There are five HCUP databases or collections of databases: the *State Inpatient Databases* (SID), the *State Ambulatory Surgery Databases* (SASD), the *State Emergency Department Databases* (SEDD), the *Nationwide Inpatient Sample* (NIS), and the *Kids' Inpatient Database* (KID). State participation in the HCUP is voluntary: thirty-seven states were included in 2003, although not all participated in every aspect. Nonetheless, the HCUP represents the largest collection of data regarding all-payer (including Medicaid, Medicare, private insurance, and the uninsured), inpatient, ED, and ambulatory surgery available for the United States.

Focus

The SID is a collection of databases containing all the discharge records from included hospitals in participating states. Each state's SID is stored in a separate file and may include unique elements, as well as certain data elements collected by all states, which are edited and recoded by AHRQ so all state files use the same structure and coding scheme for the common data elements. Common data elements in the SID include patient demographics, expected payment source, patient charges, length of stay, diagnoses, procedures, admission and discharge status, and hospital characteristics such as size and type of ownership. Some states include two other types of data that allow SID records to be linked to other data sources: county identifiers, which allow linkage with the Area Resource Files, and hospital identifiers, which allow linkage with the American Hospital Association database.

Two of the HCUP databases are created from probability samples of SID records. The NIS is the largest all-payer patient database in the United States; it contains information similar to the SID. The KID samples discharge records for children (defined in 2003 as persons age 20 and younger) and is the only all-payer database for inpatient care for children in the United States. The data elements included are similar to the NIS, with the addition of age in months for children younger than 10 years; designation of whether the stay was for an uncomplicated birth in the hospital; and a field designating the hospital as a children's general hospital, children's specialty hospital, children's unit in a general hospital, or not a children's hospital.

The SEDD contain information from participating states about ED visits that do not result in hospitalization; visits that do result in hospitalization are included in the SID. As with the SID, data from each state are stored separately, and the files are edited by AHRQ for uniformity, although unique data elements remain in the files from some states. Types of data collected in the SEDD are similar to that collected by the NIS. Currently, thirteen states participate in the SEDD, and of those, three make their files available to outside researchers.

The SASD are a set of databases that contains information on ambulatory surgeries performed in participating states. Ambulatory surgery is defined as surgery performed on the same day a patients is admitted and released. In some states, information from freestanding surgery centers, as well as from surgery sites affiliated with hospitals, is included. As with the SID and SEDD, each state's information is stored in a separate file and, although some data elements are common to all states and have been edited for uniformity, each state's files may also contain unique elements. Information available from the SASD is similar to that captured in the NIS. Currently, twenty states participated in the SASD.

Data Collection

Every state that participates in HCUP contributes at least its state's discharge records to the SID, making the SID the largest of the state-specific databases and the source of the records sampled for the NIS and KID. The SID, SEDD, and SASD include all discharge records from states who participate. They are therefore censuses rather than samples. For most states, the SID contains all records from all community hospitals in the state. However, in some states, private data organizations provide the SID data and only include data from their member hospitals. Information about the inclusiveness of SID data is available in the SID technical documentation.

Data for the NIS and KID are selected from the hospitals included in the SID, using probability sampling so the data may be weighted to create nationally valid estimates of hospital utilization. The NIS is based on a stratified sample of hospitals included in the HCUP; all patient discharge records for the year are included for a hospital that is selected for the sample. Each year about 1000 hospitals are sampled, and 5 to 8 million patient records are included. The sampling frame in 2003 included about 90 percent of all hospital discharges, and the sample represents about 20 percent of all community hospitals. The KID sample is drawn using stratification similar to that of the NIS, with the addition of a hospital identifier for children's hospitals. In 2003, the KID included discharge records from 3438 hospitals in thirty-six states.

Accessing Data and Ancillary Materials

HCUP data are available for purchase from the "HCUP Central Distributor" page of the AHRQ website (http://www.hcup-us.ahrq.gov/tech/assist/centdist.jsp). Prospective users must submit an application to AHRQ and must agree to not use the data for commercial purposes or to identify individual respondents. In general, HCUP data files are available on CD-ROM in ASCII format, and the CD-ROM includes documentation and SAS and SPSS syntax files to convert the ASCII files to either format. NIS data are available for the years 1988 to 2003. For the years 1993 to 2000, each year's data are sold separately on a single CD-ROM, whereas data for the years 1988 to 1992 must be purchased as a six–CD-ROM set. KID data are available for the years 1997, 2000, and 2003, and data for each year may be purchased separately.

Availability of the state-level databases (the SID, SASD, and SEDD) is considerably more complicated because each state's data are stored in a separate file, and different states have participated in different years.

In addition, each state sets the price for access to its data: for 2003, data prices ranged from $20 to $3170. SID data are available for the years 1990 to 2004; SASD data for 1997, 1998, 1999, 2000, 2001, 2002, 2003, and 2004; and SEDD for 1999, 2000, 2001, 2002, 2003, and 2004. Detailed information about availability and price for the state-level databases is available from the HCUP Central Distributor web page referenced previously.

It is also possible to access SID, NIS, and KID data and perform simple analyses without purchasing the data, by using HCUPnet, a free web-based query system available at http://hcup.ahrq.gov/HCUPnet.asp. HCUPnet offers separate interfaces for both novice and expert users. Both interfaces allow the user to create queries by checking options on a series of lists, ultimately creating frequency tables or rank-ordered lists such as the ten most common principal diagnoses in 2003.

The Medical Expenditures Panel Survey

The MEPS is conducted by the AHRQ to collect information on health care utilization and costs in the United States. It allows the calculation of valid estimates of health care costs, utilization, and insurance coverage, and access at the national level and within the four Census regions (Northeast, Midwest, South, and West). The MEPS consists of four components: the *Household Component* (HC), the *Nursing Home Component* (NHC), the *Medical Provider Component* (MPC), and the *Insurance Component* (IC). Of these, only the HC data are publicly available. NHC and MPC data may be used at the AHRQ's Center for Financing, Access, and Cost Trends Data Center, and the IC data may be accessed through the MPHSnet online interface.

Focus

The MEPS HC is a survey that collects data on all members of a sampled household or family. Topics covered by the HC include family demographics; health conditions; health status; health care utilization, including hospital stays, ED and OPD visits, physician visits, dental care, home health care, prescription and over-the-counter medications, and other medical expenses; health care charges and payments; health insurance; household income and assets; and employment. The NHC, which was conducted in 1996 only, gathered information from a sample of nursing homes and residents. Information gathered from facilities included size, ownership, and staffing. Information gathered from residents included demographics, medical conditions, health status, and insurance. The MPC collects data from hospitals, physicians, and home health care providers. It includes information that can be used to estimate the expenses of people enrolled in managed care plans. The IC consists of two parts: the household sample and the list sample. The household sample is a survey of respondents to the HC and collects detailed information on insurance offered to, and held by, members of those households. The list sample gathers information about the amount, types, and costs of health insurance available from employers, through a survey of a sample of business establishments and governments in the United States.

Data Collection

The HC has been conducted since 1996 on a nationally representative sample of the civilian, noninstitutionalized U.S. population. Response rates have been in the 65 to 70 percent range each year. The HC uses an overlapping panel design so each sampled household is included in the HC for 2 full calendar years. The HC sampling frame is drawn from the previous year's NHIS, and it is possible to link records from the MEPS to records in the NHIS. HC data are collected from a single member of a household, who provides information about all family and household members.

The NHC was conducted only in 1996, on a nationally representative sample of nursing homes and residents of nursing homes. Data collected about the facilities include ownership, staffing, number of beds, number of residents, type and size of special care units, and structure (i.e., if it was part of a hospital or retirement center). Data collected from residents include demographics, insurance coverage, health status, and medical conditions. The residents' data file can be linked to the facilities data file, and the sample design allows for the production of person-level estimates while controlling for facility-level characteristics, although it is not possible to use the linked file to produce facility-level estimates while controlling for person-level characteristics.

The MPC is a survey conducted with hospitals, physicians, and medical providers working under their supervision, as well as home health care agencies, long-term care institutions, and other medical facilities who provided care to individuals included in the HC. These data are collected only if the HC respondent gives consent to have MEPS contact his or her care providers. MPC data are collected the year following that when the care was received, with the purpose of verifying and supplementing information provided in the HC about charges, payments, and sources of payment for health services. MPC data are used to edit and impute values on the HC and are not based on a nationally representative sample, so it is not released as a stand-alone data file.

The IC has been conducted annually since 1996, although the composition of the population sampled has changed several times. The IC collects data on employer-based health insurance, including the number of employers offering insurance, characteristics of those employers, cost of the insurance, the number of people enrolled, and characteristics of available health plans. IC data were originally collected from two different samples: the household sample and the list sample. The *household sample* was originally selected from the insurance providers (unions and insurance companies) and employers of respondents to the previous year's HC. These providers and employers acted as proxy respondents who provided insurance information for the HC respondents. The data collected were then attached to the respondent's HC record. After 1996, self-employed individuals and insurance companies were dropped from the IC, and insurance offered directly from unions was dropped in 1997. Although data were collected 1996, 1997, 1998, 1999, 2001, and 2002, data collection from the IC household sample has been discontinued. The *list sample* is drawn from lists of private and public employers, and provides a nationally representative sample of workplaces. Data collected through the list sample include health plans offered, enrollment, and costs.

Accessing Data and Ancillary Materials

MEPS HC data for the years 1996 to 2004 are available for download from the MEPS data site; they may also be ordered from MEPS or, for a fee, from the NTIS. HC data for a given year are released in a number of separate data files, of which there are five types: person-level files, event-level files, condition-level files, job-level files, and person-round-policyholder-establishment–level files. Two sources of information to help disentangle this information are available on the MEPS website: the HC FAQ, and the matrices known as "Variable Locators," which organize variables by concept, analysis level, and file number. HC data are available in ASCII and SAS transport formats; ancillary materials available include detailed documentation about the survey, a codebook, and SAS and SPSS syntax.

Data from the NHC and MPC components are not publicly accessible because of confidentiality restrictions and the nonrepresentative nature of the MPC sample. However, researchers may apply for access to this data at the AHRQ's Center for Financing, Access, and Cost Trends Data Center. Data from the IC are not available because of confidentiality restrictions, except for the years in which IC information was linked to HC records. However, the MEPSnet online interface allows the user to produce tables using IC data.

A number of MEPS survey instruments are available for download from the "Survey Questionnaires – Household Component" and "Survey Questionnaires – Insurance Component" pages of the MEPS website (http://www.meps.ahrq.gov/mepsweb/survey_comp/survey.jsp and http://www.meps.ahrq.gov/mepsweb/survey_comp/survey_ic.jsp, respectively). A bibliography of reports and papers using MEPS data, some with links to the text of the publication, is available from the "Publications" section of the MEPS website at http://www.meps.ahrq.gov/mepsweb/data_stats/publications.jsp.

MEPSnet is an online, menu-driven data analysis interface that allows users to create tables and compute simple statistics using HC and IC data. Data are available for the years 1996 to 1999, and available analytic options include frequencies, cross-tabulations, means, minima, maxima, sums, medians, and ratios.

The National Immunization Survey

The NIS collects data on childhood immunization rates for children living in the United States. The NIS began collecting data in 1994, and allows the estimation of up-to-date immunization levels nationally and in each state, the District of Columbia, and twenty-seven large urban areas. The NIS is conducted by the National Opinion Research Center for the CDC; it is jointly sponsored by the National Immunization Program and the NCHS.

Focus

The NIS began as part of the Childhood Immunization Initiative (CII), established in 1992. The CII has a number of goals relating to immunization, including reducing costs to parents, improving delivery of vaccines to children, enhancing awareness and community participation, and monitoring vaccination coverage. The NIS was established to serve the latter objective and, subsequently, has also served the purpose of measuring progress toward other immunization goals such as those stated in *Healthy People 2000* and *Healthy People 2010.*

Data Collection

The target population of the NIS is children between the ages of 19 and 35 months living in the United States at the time of the survey. Data about these children's immunizations are collected from a parent or other adult from the child's household who is knowledgeable about the child's immunization record. If possible, data are also collected from the child's immunization providers. NIS data are collected by telephone interview, and the sample of households is selected using random-digit-dial technology. If a selected household contains a child in the target age range, a telephone interview is conducted to collect information from the parent or other knowledgeable household member about immunizations the child has received, the dates of the immunizations, and demographic and socioeconomic information about the household. If the parent or guardian grants permission, the child's vaccination providers are contacted by mail to verify the child's vaccination record; this phase of the survey is called the Provider Record Check (PRC).

The vaccinations included in the NIS are those recommended by the Advisory Committee on Immunization Practices. The current recommendations are currently four doses of diphtheria, tetanus, and acellular pertussis vaccine; three doses of polio vaccine; measles/mumps/rubella vaccine; *Haemophilus influenzae* type b vaccine; hepatitis A vaccine (Hep A); three doses of hepatitis B vaccine; varicella zoster vaccine (chickenpox); four doses of pneumococcal conjugate vaccine (PCV); and influenza vaccine. Hep A is recommended only in selected states with a high incidence of that disease. All vaccines except varicella, influenza, and PCV have been included in the NIS since its inception. PCV was added in 2002, and influenza and Hep A were added in 2003.

Nonvaccination information collected in the telephone interview portion of the NIS includes the child's date of birth, gender, race, and Hispanic origin; if a shot card (paper record of the vaccines) is available, the vaccines the child has had and their dates; if no shot card is available, information about the number of and each type of vaccine; number of adults and children residing in the household; income; household place of residence at the child's birth; respondent's relationship to the child; and the mother's marital status, race, Hispanic origin, and education. If the parent or guardian grants permission, the name(s) and contact information for the children's vaccination provider(s) are also collected to administer the PRC.

The PRC data are collected from mail questionnaires sent to each provider for whom the parent has granted permission to contact. In 2004, 30,987 children were included in the household interview portion of the NIS, while 21,998 had "adequate provider data," meaning that sufficient vaccination history information could be gathered from their providers to determine if they were up to date with their vaccinations.

Accessing Data and Ancillary Materials

Currently, NIS data for the years 1995 to 2004 are available for download from the NIS website (http://www.cdc.gov/nis/datafiles.htm). Each year's data are stored in a separate data file, in ASCII format. Ancillary information available for each year includes a *User's Guide*, which provides detailed information about the sampling plan and variance estimation, a codebook, and SAS syntax to translate the ASCII file to an SAS data set and add variable formats.

The Surveillance Epidemiology and End Results Program

The SEER program collects information on cancer incidence, treatment, and survival from a number of population-based cancer registries in the United States. Although SEER data do not represent a probability sample of cancer patients in the United States, the geographic area covered does include 26 percent of the U.S. population. In addition, that area has been expanded in recent years to include more members of underrepresented minority groups.

Focus

The SEER program of the National Cancer Institute (NCI) was established as part of the National Cancer Act of 1971, which had as its goal the collection, analysis, and dissemination of information useful in the prevention, diagnosis, and treatment of cancer. Specific goals of the SEER program include creating periodic estimates of cancer incidence and mortality, monitoring annual cancer incidence trends for changes in occurrence in population subgroups (e.g., in a particular racial group or geographic area), providing information on changes over time in cancer therapies and survival rates, and promoting studies to identify factors related to cancer such as occupational exposures and early detection practices. The SEER program is currently funded by a combination of the NCI, the CDC (through the National Program of Cancer Registries), and the individual states.

Data Collection

SEER data are collected from cancer registries in the United States. Although geographic coverage has changed over the years, SEER has always included information on all cancers diagnosed among residents of the geographic areas included at a particular time. The program began in 1973 with data from Connecticut, Iowa, New Mexico, Utah, Hawaii, and the metropolitan areas of Detroit and San Francisco/Oakland. Metropolitan Atlanta and the Seattle–Puget Sound area were added in 1974 to 1975. In 1978, ten predominantly African American counties in rural Georgia were added, and in 1980, data from Native Americans in Arizona was added. New Orleans, New Jersey, and Puerto Rico also participated for parts of the 1970s and/or 1980s. In 1992, Los Angeles County and four counties in the San Jose/Monterey area south of San Francisco were added to increase Hispanic representation. A registry for Alaska Natives is also currently included. In 2001, Kentucky and the remaining counties in California were added, and New Jersey and Louisiana resumed participation.

The SEER population (i.e., the population living in the geographic areas included in SEER) is similar to the U.S. population in poverty and education, slightly more urban, and more likely to be foreign born. Most racial minorities are overrepresented: for instance, 40 percent of U.S. Hispanics, 42 percent of Native Americans and Alaska Natives, 53 percent of Asians, and 70 percent of Hawaiian/Pacific Islanders are included in the SEER population.

NCI staff work with the North American Association of Central Cancer Registries to provide expertise and guidance to assure data quality and comparability so data from the registries may be pooled to create national estimates. The SEER program also provides computer software (SEER*Stat) that allows users to access SEER data and perform computations such as calculating incidence-based mortality rates.

Information collected by SEER includes the name of the registry; the cancer patient's place of birth, year of birth, race and ethnicity, gender, and age and marital status at diagnosis; date of diagnosis; primary site of tumor; laterality of tumor; histologic type of tumor; grade of tumor; whether surgical treatment was used; whether radiation treatment was used; and vital status of patient.

Accessing Data and Ancillary Materials

SEER data are updated annually. The current file covers the years 1973 to 2003. Public-use SEER files are available in several formats, and both SEER data and SEER*Stat, a software package created by NCI to facilitate use of SEER data, are available free of charge. To access the SEER public-use data, however, the researcher must first submit a Public-Use Data Agreement. A copy of this form required is available on the SEER website at http://seer.cancer.gov/publicdata/options.html. This site also contains information regarding how to request or download the data files and documentation. Four methods may be used to access the SEER public-use data:

1. Download and install SEER*Stat on your computer, and then access SEER data through an Internet connection. This option allows data analysis only using SEER*Stat.
2. Request SEER data and SEER*Stat on CD-ROM, and install the data and software on your computer. The first CD in this set includes a binary file of SEER data plus SEER*Stat; the second includes the ASCII version of the SEER data, which may be analyzed using any statistical program (e.g., SAS or SPSS).
3. Request SEER*Stat and the SEER data on DVD; this content is identical to that contained the CD set described previously.
4. Download the CD image files from the Internet; this content is identical to the CD described previously. If you will only access the data using SEER*Stat, you need to download only the first CD image file.

Files linking SEER data with Medicare data were first created in 1991 and have been updated in 1995, 1999, and 2003. In the future, these files are slated for update every 3 years. In these files, the records of persons age 65 and older in the SEER files are linked to their Medicare records when possible. This has been successful about 93 percent of the time. Although personal identifiers have been removed from these files, they are not public-use files because of the possibility of identifying an individual through a combination of variables such as age, race, and type of tumor. Further information about the process to be followed in requesting SEER-Medicare files, as well as the costs involved, are available from the NCI website at http://healthservices.cancer.gov/seermedicare/obtain/.

Health Behaviors and Risk Factors Data

This chapter discusses three major surveys that collect data regularly and at a national level on health behaviors and behavioral risks to health in the United States. The *Behavioral Risk Factor Surveillance System* (BRFSS) collects data annually from community-dwelling adults (age 18 and older) on a broad range of health behaviors and risks. The *Youth Risk Behavior Surveillance System* (YRBSS) collects data on a smaller number of risk factors in odd-numbered years from ninth- through twelfth-grade students. *Monitoring the Future* (MTF) collects data annually and focuses on the use and abuse of alcohol, tobacco, and drugs among students attending the eighth, tenth, and twelfth grades. It also collects data in an ongoing follow-up study of a sample of students originally included in the MTF sample as twelfth-graders.

The Behavioral Risk Factor Surveillance System

The BRFSS is a survey of behavioral risks to health among American adults conducted annually by the CDC in cooperation with state health departments. Preliminary surveys were conducted in the years 1981 to 1983, and the BRFSS officially began collecting data in 1984 with fifteen states participating. Since 1994, all fifty states, the District of Columbia, and the territories of Puerto Rico, Guam, and the U.S. Virgin Islands have been included in the BRFSS.

Focus

The primary focus of the BRFSS is collecting data on individual health and health risk behaviors, using sampling techniques that allow accurate estimates of those behaviors at the state and national levels. The BRFSS was developed in response to the growing awareness among epidemiologists and public health officials of the influence that individual health and health risk behaviors such as smoking and exercise exerted on morbidity and mortality. In the early 1980s, there was no coordinated national effort to collect data on individual health and health risk behaviors, so the BRFSS was developed to meet that need.

Another important purpose of the BRFSS is to guide and evaluate public health efforts at the state level. This is a reflection of the fact that in the United States, much of the responsibility for monitoring public health, as well as developing and evaluating public health interventions, lies at the state level rather than at the national level. This emphasis is clear in several aspects of the BRFSS, including the fact that the survey itself is conducted through a partnership with the CDC and the state health departments, that individual states can partially customize the BRFSS questionnaire to collect data that they view as particularly important within their state, and that data are collected and weighted so they can be used to make accurate estimates of the prevalence of different behaviors and health conditions for each state. Some states also stratify their samples to allow them to estimate prevalence for specific metropolitan areas or regions within the state.

The BRFSS questionnaire used in a given year consists of three parts:

1. The *core component,* which consists of questions asked with standard wording and in a standard order in all states and territories
2. *Optional modules,* consisting of questions on a number of topics that are developed by the CDC and that a given state can choose whether to administer; although once chosen, the module must be administered in its entirety and exactly as written
3. *State-added questions,* which are developed or otherwise acquired by an individual state in response to the state's specific concerns

The core component is further divided into *fixed* core component questions, which are asked every year; *rotating* core component questions, which are asked every other year; and *emerging issues* core questions, which typically focus on late-breaking health issues. Topics covered by fixed core questions include demographic information and major health risks such as smoking. Rotating core questions are included as optional modules in years that they are not included as core questions and cover many topics, including health conditions such as arthritis and diabetes and health risks such as smokeless tobacco use and exposure to firearms. As many as ten questions on emerging issues can be included in the core in a given year. After that year, they are evaluated and are either discontinued or incorporated into either the core or optional modules.

Optional modules consist of a number of questions focused on a particular topic. For instance, in 2005, there were twenty-six optional modules on a range of topics, including diabetes, prostate cancer screening, indoor air quality, weight control, and intimate partner violence.

State-added questions are chosen by an individual state and included in the BRFSS at the state's own expense. The BRFSS does not develop or supervise these questions, and data from state-added questions are not stored on the BRFSS website. However, lists of state-added questions, by state and by category, for the years 1998 to 2002 are available on the BRFSS website. State-added questions can deal with different subjects than those included in the core and module components of the BRFSS, gather data on core or module topics in greater detail, or include topics in years that are not included in the core or module of the main BRFSS. Topics covered by state-added questions in 2002, for instance, included birth control, colorectal cancer screening, gambling, oral health, and sexual behavior. Inquiries about state-added questions and data gathered from them should be addressed to the BRFSS coordinator for the state in question. A list of state coordinators is available on the BRFSS website at http://www2.cdc.gov/nccdphp/brfss2/coordinator.asp.

Data Collection

BRFSS data are collected through telephone surveys of community-dwelling adults older than 18 years. Persons living in institutions or who do not have telephones are automatically excluded from participation. Currently, households are selected through random-digit-dialing, and one adult in a selected household is surveyed. BRFSS data are gathered on a rolling basis throughout the year by state health departments or by contractors such as a university survey research center, using a standardized questionnaire developed by the CDC. The states send the collected data to the CDC, who aggregates the data, returns it to the state, and publishes it on the CDC website.

BRFSS data are collected using sampling procedures and weighted so accurate estimates of risk behaviors can be made at the state and national levels. In 2005, all states and two territories used a disproportionate stratified sample design, while Puerto Rico and the U.S. Virgin islands used a simple random sample design. In either case, the different weighting factors are combined into a single variable (*FINALWT* in 2005) that can be used to weight the data to represent the population of noninstitutionalized adults older than 18 years.

Accessing Data and Ancillary Materials

BRFSS data files and ancillary materials such as codebooks and questionnaires are available for free download from the BRFSS website. In general, BRFSS data files and supporting materials are stored by year. For instance, the 2005 data, codebook, technical reports, and SAS syntax files are all available for download from the same web page. The primary exception is questionnaires and information about questions included by state and year, which must be accessed from a different section of the website.

BRFSS data sets and most ancillary information can be accessed through the "Technical Information and Data" page of the BRFSS website (http://www.cdc.gov/brfss/technical_infodata/surveydata.htm). For 2005 data, available ancillary materials included an overview of the BRFSS (which includes a description of the data collection and cleaning process), the codebook, explanations of calculated variables, and lists of optional modules used, by state and by category. Data files for 2005 are available in ASCII and SAS Transport formats, and SAS syntax and format files are included to convert the ASCII or SAS Transport data files to an SAS data file and to add formats to it.

Further technical information is contained in the *BRFSS Policy Memos* (a.k.a. "*Numbered Memos*") from the years 1993 to 2003 and the *Summary Data Quality Reports* for the years 1998 to 2004. Both are available from the main "Technical Information and Data" page of the BRFSS website.

BRFSS questionnaires, produced in both English and Spanish since 1997, are available for download through the "Questionnaires" page of the website (http://www.cdc.gov/brfss/questionnaires/questionnaires. htm). This page also includes an index of optional modules used, by state and category, for the years 1998 to 2005, and an index of state-added questions, by state and category, for the years 1998 to 2002. BRFSS questions are generally in the public domain and can be used without permission.

Researchers interested in data on particular subjects, rather than particular years, can approach the BRFSS through the "Historical Questions" page of the BRFSS website (http://apps.nccd.cdc.gov/brfssQuest/). This page includes an interface that allows searching for questions in broad categories or through a free-text search for particular words, for the years 1985 to 2003. The search results include the exact text of questions matching the subject or words in question, the year asked, and whether the questions were core or optional. For instance, a search on the topic "Social Context" reveals that five questions on this subject were included in optional modules in the years 1996 to 1999. They asked about perceived safety, home ownership, length of time at current residence, emotional support, and food security. A text search on the term "condom" returned twenty questions, some core and some module, from the years 1992 to 2003. The topic interface allows you to determine in which years questions pertaining to a particular subject were included. Having determined that, you can proceed to the "Technical Information and Data" page of the BRFSS website and download the data and supporting materials for the year or years in question.

The CDC website provides an online menu-driven interface that allows the computation of prevalence data by topic, state, and year, without requiring the user to download data. Only a limited number of questions are available through this interface, which returns the sample size, point estimate, and confidence interval and creates a bar chart for a specific question. A similar interface for trend analysis for the years 1990 to 2002 is also available, as is an interface for data from metropolitan areas, for the years 2002 to 2004. Finally, a limited mapping facility (for the national level only) is available for 2004 data. These options can be accessed from the index on the BRFSS "Prevalence Data" page (http://apps.nccd.cdc.gov/brfss/).

The "Publications and Research" page of the BRFSS website (http://www.cdc.gov/brfss/pubs/index.htm) includes links to a number of full-text reports based on BRFSS data, information about research initiatives, a bibliography of methodologic publications based on or relating to the BRFSS, and links to searchable databases of scientific publications, state publications, and *Morbidity and Mortality Weekly Reports* issues based on BRFSS data.

The Youth Risk Behavior Surveillance System

The YRBSS was developed in 1990 to study health risk behaviors among young people in the United States. It is conducted every 2 years, in odd-numbered years, during the spring semester (February–May), on nationally representative samples of students enrolled in the ninth through twelfth grades. The YRBSS targets six categories of behavior: tobacco use, alcohol, and drug use; behaviors that contribute to unintentional injuries and violence; unsafe sexual behaviors; dietary behaviors; and physical activity. It remains the only nationally representative survey conducted regularly in the United States that gathers information about youth health risk behaviors.

Focus

The principal focus of the YRBSS is health risk behaviors among young adults, in particular, those behaviors that are believed to be adopted and become established during childhood and adolescence. The YRBSS was developed partly in response to the increasing awareness in the 1980s of the importance of individual risk behaviors on morbidity and mortality. This awareness led to the establishment of the BRFSS, which collects data on health risk behaviors from persons age 18 and older. The YRBSS was developed, in part, to gather similar information regarding the prevalence of health risk behaviors among young people. Like the BRFSS, the YRBSS is also constructed to allow the assessment of trends in risk behavior over time, the cooccurrence of multiple risk behaviors, and the differences in risk behaviors among subgroups. However, the YRBSS focuses on a smaller set of risk behaviors, and specifically on concrete behaviors, rather than determinants of those behaviors such as beliefs and attitudes.

The YRBSS includes national, state, and local surveys. The national survey is conducted by the CDC and provides nationally representative data on high school students. The state and local surveys, conducted by departments of health and education, provide data representative of the state or local school district where they were conducted. Three other national surveys are included within the YRBSS: the *Youth Behavior Survey*, the *National College Health Risk Behavior Survey*, and the *National Alternative High School Youth Risk Behavior Survey*. The Youth Risk Behavior Survey was a follow-back survey to the National Health Interview Survey (NHIS) and was conducted in 1992 among approximately 10,465 young people age 12 to 21 years. In contrast to the YRBSS, students not attending school were also included in the sample. The National College Health Risk Behavior Survey was a mail survey administered to a representative sample of 4609 students attending 2- and 4-year colleges in 1995. The National Alternative High School Youth Risk Behavior Survey was conducted in 1998 among a representative sample of approximately 9000 students attending alternative high schools. Special population surveys, for instance, of Navajo youth, have also been conducted periodically.

Data Collection

The same questionnaire is used for all YRBSS survey sites in a given year. The questionnaire is revised before each biennial survey, with input from the CDC, states, and local school districts. Although the YRBSS focus remains on the six categories of subjects enumerated previously, questions on other topics can also be included in a particular administration. For instance, the 2005 questionnaire included two questions about asthma. The YRBSS is a pencil-and-paper survey that is self-administered by students who record their responses on a computer-scannable answer sheet or booklet. It is completed at the student's school during a normal class period. For the national survey and most state and local surveys, trained data collectors supervise questionnaire administration, and record information about the grade level and size of the sampled classes. Some state and local surveys are administered by teachers of the selected classes. In either case, the data collector or teacher introduces the survey and reads the instructions using a standardized script. Most data cleaning and editing of YRBSS data are performed by Westat and the CDC.

The national YRBSS uses a cluster sample design with three stages:

1. Counties or groups of counties are the PSUs
2. Schools are selected within PSUs
3. One or two classes are selected within each school, and all students within a sampled class are selected

Black and Hispanic students are oversampled. This is corrected with a sampling weight assigned to each respondent, based on gender, race/ethnicity, and school grade. Response rates since 1991 have ranged from 75 to 81 percent for schools and 83 to 90 percent for students.

State and local surveys use a two-stage cluster sample design. In most cases, only public schools are included: (1) schools are selected, generally with a probability proportional to their enrollment, and (2) intact classes are selected randomly by subject or during a fixed time period (e.g., third period classes).

Usually, the sampling frame is defined by school district rather than the metropolitan area. Weighting is applied to state and local surveys that use scientific sampling procedures, provide information about those procedures, and have a response rate greater than 60 percent. In these surveys, the weights can be used to calculate statistics that are representative of students attending grades nine through twelve in the relevant jurisdiction. Surveys with a response rate of less than 60 percent or that do not provide information about their sample selection procedures are not weighted and thus cannot be used to generalize beyond the specific students surveyed. In 2003, thirty-two states and twenty districts had weighted data, while eleven states and two districts did not.

Although data are collected from individual students within certain classes in particular schools, most geographic and demographic information is suppressed in the publicly available YRBSS data sets because of confidentiality concerns. Schools are identified in the publicly available data only by large Census geographic region (Northeast, Midwest, South, or West) and by metropolitan status, and only limited demographic information about students is available, such as age, grade, gender, race/ethnicity, height, and weight. Not every state is included in every year the YRBSS has been conducted. For instance, in 2003, the states of Washington, Minnesota, and Virginia did not participate at all, while only selected regions of California, Pennsylvania, and Delaware participated. Therefore, 2003 data from the last three states can be used to produce estimates of only the metropolitan areas that participated in the YRBSS.

Accessing Data and Ancillary Materials

National YRBSS data for the years 1991, 1993, 1995, 1997, 1997, 2001, 2003 and 2005 are available for download from the "National Data Files & Documentation 1991–2005" page of the YRBSS website (http://www.cdc. gov/HealthyYouth/yrbs/data/index.htm). Data and ancillary information are stored separately for each year. YRBSS data are available in ASCII, SPSS, and SAS formats, and an SAS formats file is also available for each year. A document presenting introductory information about the YRBSS, including a codebook and description of the data collection procedures and weighting methods used, is also provided for each year of data. The data and ancillary materials for the National College Health Risk Behavior Survey (1995) and the National Alternative High School Youth Risk Behavior Survey (1998) are also available for download from this web page. The YRBSS questionnaire, for 2005 only, is available from the main YRBSS website (http://www.cdc.gov/HealthyYouth/yrbs/index.htm).

The "Youth Online: Comprehensive Results" page of the YRBSS website (http://apps.nccd.cdc.gov/yrbss/) includes a menu-based interface that allows the user to display point estimates and confidence intervals for the prevalence of a risk factor, nationally or by state, for 1 or more years.

The main YRBSS web page includes links to a number of reports based on YRBSS data, a bibliography of research using YRBSS data, a document explaining the rationale for the inclusion of specific questions in the 2005 questionnaire, and a detailed *Morbidity and Mortality Weekly Report* article from 2004 on the history and methodology of the YRBSS.

Monitoring the Future

The MTF is an annual survey of the attitudes, values, and behaviors of a nationally representative sample of American high school students and young adults. It is conducted by the Survey Research Center of the University of Michigan, with funding from the National Institute on Drug Abuse of the National Institutes of Health (NIH). MTF began collecting data, originally on twelfth-graders (high school seniors) only, in 1975; since 1991, eighth- and tenth-graders have also been surveyed. Currently, approximately 50,000 students in the eighth, tenth, and twelfth grades are surveyed each year; young people of similar ages who are not attending school are not included in the survey. Although the main MTF survey is cross-sectional, it also has a longitudinal aspect in that a randomly selected sample of students from each senior class is chosen for follow-up surveys. Students selected for the longitudinal sample are sent follow-up mail questionnaires every other year on a continuing basis.

Focus

The primary focus of MTF is the use and abuse of tobacco, alcohol, and drugs by young adults, and their perceptions and attitudes toward these substances. The MTF consists of two parts: (1) core questions that include demographic information and basic questions about substance use that are asked of every respondent, and (2) ancillary questions on a variety of topics such as social and political attitudes, health behaviors, and educational aspirations, which are administered to different subsamples of respondents through the use of six different questionnaire forms. These questionnaire forms are referred to in the MTF data archives as Forms 1 through 6. This structure allows MTF to collect data that allow detailed and precise estimates of the prevalence of substance use behaviors in young people, while also collecting data on a broad range of topics related to their general well-being.

The core section of the 2004 MTF included 207 questions. Many were concerned with substance use and abuse, including a series of questions about the frequency of use of a number of substances in the last 30 days, in the last year, and over the respondent's lifetime. Substances covered in this section of the 2004 MTF include tobacco, alcohol, LSD, hashish, amphetamines, Quaaludes, methamphetamine, cocaine, heroin, ecstasy, and Ritalin. Other core questions in 2004 concerned political beliefs, religious behavior, educational aspirations, intended military service, employment and income, recreation, and automobile driving, including accidents and driving while intoxicated or under the influence of a drug.

Questions included in Forms 1 through 6 generally ask about issues related to those in the core, or ask more detailed questions about the same topics. For instance, a core question in 2004 asked how often the respondent "went out for fun and recreation" in a typical week, while Form 1 included a series of questions about how often a respondent went to the movies, attended a rock concert, or went driving or motorcycle riding for fun. A detailed chart of questions included in MTF by year is provided in the *User's Guide* available on the ICPSR website for each MTF data set.

Data Collection

Most of the data collected by MTF are gathered through an annual cross-sectional survey of students currently attending school in the eighth, tenth, or twelfth grades. These data are collected through self-administered questionnaires completed by individual students, usually during a normal class period at their school. The survey administration is supervised by University of Michigan staff members, and data are not shared with either the students' parents or school officials. Questionnaire forms are optically scanned and stored as an electronic data file.

MTF uses a probability sample design with three selection stages:

1. Census broad geographic area (Northeast, Midwest, South, or West)
2. Schools or linked groups of schools within a broad geographic area
3. Students within schools – if a school has less than 350 students in the relevant grade, all are selected; if there are more than 350, participants are randomly selected

Schools who decline to participate are replaced with schools similar in type (public, Catholic, or private/non-Catholic), geographic location, and size. Specific questionnaire forms (six were used in 2004) are administered in an ordered sequence so a nearly identical subsample of students completes each form. About 1400 questions were administered in total, of which about one-third are core demographic and substance use questions administered to all students; the other questions are divided across the six forms and thus administered to only a sample of the students. Participation rate has been 66 to 85 percent throughout the study.

A longitudinal component was added to the MTF in 1976. Since then, a random sample of about 2400 students from that year's twelfth-grade participants has been selected to participate in follow-up surveys. These participants are divided into two groups and are mailed questionnaires in alternating years so half the participants receive a questionnaire in odd-numbered years following twelfth grade (i.e., years 1, 3, 5, and so on), while half receive follow-up questionnaires in even-numbered years. Retention for the first year of follow-up averages 77 percent.

Accessing Data and Ancillary Materials

MTF data and ancillary information are available for download through the website of the ICPSR (http://webapp.icpsr.umich.edu/cocoon/ ICPSR-SERIES/00035.xml). Each year of data is stored separately, and within a given year data are divided into that collected from twelfth-graders versus that collected from eighth- and tenth-graders. There is a further subdivision by questionnaire form. For instance, in 2004, there are seven separate files for twelfth-graders: one containing responses to the core questions, and one for responses to each of the forms used to administer the questions asked of only a subsample of participants. MTF data are available in SAS, SPSS, Stata, and ASCII formats, and SAS, SPSS, and Stata syntax files are available to perform tasks such as adding variable and value labels. Other supporting materials available for download from the ICPSR website include a file manifest, codebook, *User's Guide*, and bibliography of research reports and articles based on MTF data.

Online analysis of MTF data is available on the ICPSR website through Survey Documentation and Analysis (SDA), a system developed by the Computer-assisted Survey Methods Program at the University of California at Berkeley. This system provides a menu-driven online interface through the "Substance Abuse and Mental Health Data Archive" page of the ICPSR website (http://www.icpsr.umich.edu/SAMHDA/ das.html) that allows researchers to access MTF data and perform basic analytic tasks without downloading data. Available statistical procedures include production of frequency and cross-tabulation tables, computation of means and standard deviations, correlations, and performance of *t* tests, analysis of variance, and multiple regression. SDA also allows users to recode and create new variables, and to download customized sets of variables and/or cases.

Data on Multiple Health Topics

This chapter discusses five surveys that gather information on multiple health-related topics. The *National Health Examination Surveys* (NHES) and its continuation, the *National Health and Nutrition Examination Survey* (NHANES), have been conducted periodically since 1960 and collect data on a wide variety of health topics through personal interview and direct physical examination. The *National Health Interview Survey* (NHIS) has been conducted annually since 1957 and gathers information through personal interviews with members of a representative sample of American households. The *Joint Canada/United States Survey of Health* (JCUSH) was conducted in 2002 to 2003, with a random sample of adults age 18 and older in Canada and the United States, was the first survey to collect comprehensive information about health and health care access in both countries. The *Longitudinal Studies of Aging* (LSOAs) consist of four surveys designed to study longitudinal changes in the health, functional status, living arrangements, and health services of older Americans as they age; the LSOAs were begun in 1984, and data were most recently collected in 2000. The *State and Local Area Integrated Telephone Survey* (SLAITS) is a data collection mechanism that has been used to conduct a number of different health-related surveys at the national, state, and local levels since 1997.

The National Health Examination Survey and the National Health and Nutrition Examination Survey

The NHES and the NHANES form part of an ongoing effort to collect data on illness and disability in the United States. This effort began in with legislative authorization in the form of the National Health Survey

Act of 1956. Both surveys use direct interview, physical examination, and laboratory testing to collect this information. The NHES was conducted three times – from 1960 to 1962, 1963 to 1965, and 1966 to 1970 – each time with a sample of approximately 7500 individuals. The NHANES has been conducted four times as a discrete study – from 1971 to 1975, 1976 to 1980, 1982 to 1984, and 1988 to 1994. In 1999, the NHANES became a continuous program that examines a nationally representative sample of about 5000 people per year.

Focus

The NHES I was conducted in 1960 to 1962 with a national probability sample of nonmilitary, noninstitutionalized adults ages 18 to 79 years. NHES I collected data on demographic characteristics, oral health, diabetes, cardiovascular disease, physical measurements, psychological distress, arthritis, and vision. Interviews were conducted with 7710 people, and physical examination information was collected for 6672 of those individuals.

NHES II was conducted from 1963 to 1965 on a national probability sample of children age 6 to 11 years. Interview data were collected from the parents of 7417 children, and physical examination data were collected on 7119 of those children. Data collected include child demographics; family composition, income, parental education, and marital status; child birth certificate data; child medical and developmental history, mother's problems during pregnancy, child developmental difficulties, and present health; school achievement, behaviors, and problems; psychological test data; overall physical health; ear, nose, and throat conditions; hearing; vision; oral health; body measurements, including height and weight; and bone age as determined from hand-wrist x-rays.

NHES III was conducted from 1966 to 1967 on a national probability sample of young people ages 12 to 17 years. Interviews were conducted with 7514 youths and their parents, and examination data were collected on 6798 of the youths. About one-third of the children examined in NHES II were included in NHES III, and it is possible to link records from NHES II and NHES III for those persons who were included in both surveys. Data collected in NHES III include youth demographics;

family income, composition, and marital status, age, race, education, and usual activity for both parents; household health episodes; youth birth certificate data; youth medical history; family decision making; personal values; school record; usual behaviors; psychological testing; body measurements; oral health; vision; ear, nose, and throat; physical examination; blood pressure; bone age; and blood testing, including screening for syphilis.

The NHANES are an extension of the NHES. In the 1970s, researchers were becoming more aware of the importance of nutrition in human health and disease, and this led to establishment of the National Nutritional Surveillance System (NNSS) under a directive from the Secretary of the Department of Health, Education and Welfare. The NNSS measured the nutritional status of the U.S. population and recorded changes in that study over time. To accomplish these goals, the NNSS was combined with the NHES to form the NHANES. Three general NHANES have been conducted and released as multiyear data sets, as well as a special survey focused on Hispanic Americans. Since 1999, the NHANES has been an annual survey, conducted continuously.

NHANES I, conducted from 1971 to 1975, and NHANES II, conducted from 1976 to 1980, used many of the same measures to allow the assessment of changes over time. In addition, both were conducted on similar age groups: NHANES I on persons age 1 to 74 years, and NHANES II on persons age 6 months to 74 years. Topics covered in NHANES I include anthropometric and biochemical measures; hearing; chest x-ray; oral health; diet; general well-being and depression; health care needs; medical history; physician's examination data; and vision. NHANES II topics included allergies; anthropometric measures; hearing; behavior; chest x-ray; health history; hematology and biochemistry; herpes and hepatitis; medical history; physician's examination data; and diet.

The *Hispanic Health and Nutrition Examination Survey* (HHANES) was conducted from 1982 to 1984. Information about the health and health behaviors of Hispanics was particularly desired at that time because this group was being recognized as a rapidly growing minority in the United States, and because NHANES I and II sampled insufficient numbers of members of Hispanics and other minority groups to estimate health and nutritional status by race or ethnicity. Data collection for HHANES was focused on the three largest Hispanic subgroups in the United States: Mexican Americans, Cuban Americans, and Puerto Ricans. It was similar in design to NHANES I and II and was conducted in regions of the country with large Hispanic populations. About 16,000 people ages 6 months to 74 years were interviewed and examined. Topics covered by HHANES included medical history; alcohol consumption; blood and urine assessments; body measurements; oral health; diabetes; diet; drug abuse; gallbladder ultrasound data; hearing; electrocardiogram data; depression; pesticide exposure; physician examination data; and vision.

NHANES III had the broadest age inclusion of any of the surveys. It included children as young as 2 months and had no upper age limit. In addition, children age 1 to 5 years and adults 60 years and older were oversampled. NHANES III included a home examination component for individuals who were unable or unwilling to come to the mobile examination center. NHANES III covered many of the same topics as NHANES I and II, and added an environmental component including data on pesticide exposure and carbon monoxide and certain trace elements in the blood. Because the NHANES went to an annual format in 1999, topics have changed somewhat each year but, as in previous years, they include demographics, diseases, medical conditions, health indicators, and risk factors such as smoking and diet. All ages are included in the annual samples.

Data Collection

All NHES and NHANES surveys collected data from both interviews and from physical examinations and laboratory testing. All but the HHANES were conducted with national probability samples that can be used, with appropriate weighting, to calculate estimates representing the American population of civilian, noninstitutionalized persons at the time of the survey for the age range included. The NHANES surveys used systematic oversampling of groups considered to be of particular interest. For instance, children and persons living below the poverty level were oversampled in both NHANES I and II because they were believed to be in particular danger of malnutrition. NHANES I also includes a subsample of adults age 25 to 74 years who were given a more detailed medical examination than were the other participants. These oversamples are corrected for in the sampling weight.

HHANES data were collected from a national sample of persons who self-reported their ethnicity or national origin as Mexican or Mexican American, Cuban or Cuban American, or Puerto Rican (including alternative terminology such as Boriucan for Puerto Rican and Chicano for Mexican). Households were selected in which at least one member described him- or herself as a member of one of these ethnic groups, and a subsampling technique was applied to select individuals within the household. The HHANES questionnaires were available in both English and Spanish, and interviews and examinations were conducted in either English or Spanish at the preference of the subject. Mexican families were sampled from the Southwest; Cubans from Dade County, Florida; and Puerto Ricans from the New York City area.

NHANES III was a much larger survey (33,994 persons) than NHANES I and II. It was based on a national probability sample with a deliberate oversampling of African Americans, Mexican Americans, young children, and older adults, to allow more precise estimates of health and nutritional factors for those groups. Since 1999, NHANES has been conducted on a continuous basis and collects data each year on a nationally representative sample of about 5000 persons. Systematic oversampling is used. For instance, the 2005 to 2006 survey oversamples adolescents age 15 to 19 years, persons age 60 and older, African Americans, and Mexican Americans, to allow more accurate estimates for those groups.

Accessing Data and Ancillary Materials

NHES data and ancillary materials are available for download from the NCHS website at http://www.cdc.gov/nchs/about/major/nhanes/cyclei_iii.htm. NHES I data are stored in eight separate files, each focused on one subject (demographics, diabetes, etc.); the files can be merged using the sequence file number that is common to the data sets. NHES I is in text format; ancillary materials include documentation, analytic guidelines, and SAS syntax to label the data and convert it to an SAS file. NHES II and NHES II data are each stored in a single text file; ancillary materials include documentation and SAS syntax to label the data and convert it to an SAS file.

NHANES I, II, and III data files and ancillary materials are available for download from the NCHS website at http://www.cdc.gov/nchs/about/major/nhanes. NHANES I, II, and III data are stored in a number of separate text files organized by topic or data source (e.g., allergy skin testing; medical history questionnaire). Ancillary materials available include documentation for each file and SAS syntax files to format and convert the data to an SAS file. HHANES data and ancillary materials are available for download from the NCHS website (http://www.cdc.gov/nchs/about/major/nhanes/hhanes.htm). HHANES data are organized in separate text files by topic or source, and ancillary information available includes documentation and SAS syntax to label the data and convert it to an SAS file. Since 1999, NHANES files include data in text format for two consecutive years. Data files are currently available for the years 1999 to 2000, 2001 to 2002, and 2003 to 2004. Ancillary materials available from this the NHANES website include the questionnaires, codebooks, and SAS syntax files to format the text data and convert it to an SAS file.

The NCHS has created data files that link the NHANES I, NHANES II, and NHANES III with the National Death Index (NDI). Only a subset of each NHANES survey is linked. In NHANES I, this subset includes only participants ages 25 to 74 years who completed a medical examination. In the NHANES II, the subset includes only participants ages 30 to 75 years who completed a medical examination, and in the NHANES III, it includes participants ages 17 and older. For NHANES I, the linked file is called the *NHANES I Epidemiological Followup Study* (NHEFS). The files thus created allow researchers to study mortality in the NHANES cohorts and to relate it to a variety of factors measured in the surveys. Further information about the linked files is available from the NCHS website (http://www.cdc.gov/nchs/r&d/nchs_datalinkage/nhefs_data_linkage_activities.htm). Because of confidentiality concerns, these linked files are not publicly available. Researchers who want to use these files must submit a proposal to the NCHS RDC. Further information about this process is available from the NCHS website at http://www.cdc.gov/nchs/about/major/nhanes/guidelines.htm.

The National Health Interview Survey

The NHIS, a survey of the health of the U.S. population, has been conducted continuously since 1957. The NHIS is conducted on a probability sample of the civilian, noninstitutionalized population living in the United States at the time of the interview and is the principal source of information about the health of that population. Content covered by the NHIS has been updated every 10 to 15 years since its inception and was substantially revised for the surveys beginning in 1997. The NHIS sampling plans have also been revised periodically; descriptions of the sample design here refer to the most recent revision, used in the years 1995 to 2004.

Focus

The NHIS began collecting data in 1957, as authorized by the National Health Survey Act of 1956, which provided for a continuing survey to collect accurate and up-to-date information on the health of the U.S. population, including the amount, distribution, and effects of illness and disability, and the health services used. It has been conducted by the NCHS since 1960, when the NCHS was formed by the combination of the National Vital Statistics Division and the National Health Survey.

In the years 1982 to 1996, the NHIS consisted of a *Core* questionnaire and one or more *Supplements*. The Core questionnaire remained stable from year to year and included basic demographic and health items. The Supplements varied from year to year, although certain Supplements, such as that pertaining to health insurance, were eventually incorporated into the NHIS Core. In 1997, the NHIS was redesigned and now consists of the three-part *Basic Module*, which is largely constant from year to year, plus *Supplements*, which vary each year. The Basic Module consists of the *Family Core*, the *Sample Adult Core*, and the *Sample Child Core*. The Family Core collects information on everyone in the family, and includes information such as household composition, basic indicators of health status, activity limitation, health insurance coverage, and health services utilization. Family Core data are maintained in five files: the Household-Level File, the Family-Level File, the Person-Level File, and two files that contain information about injuries and poisonings. The Sample

Child Core and Sample Adult Core collect more detailed information on health care services use, health status, and behavior, and are collected from one adult and one (if any) child member of each family. Different questionnaires are used for adults and children.

Currently, NHIS uses the term *Supplement* or *Supplementary Questions* to refer to questions included in the NHIS that are cosponsored with another entity such as the NCI or National Center for Injury Prevention and Control. These questions have also been referred to in the past as *Topical Modules* or *Periodic Modules*. Topics included in Supplements in the years 1997 to 2004 include immunization, mental health, use of complementary and alternative medicine, and cancer screening and sun protection. A list of topics and cosponsors is available from the NCHS website at http://www.cdc.gov/nchs/about/major/nhis/co-sponsors.htm.

Data Collection

The NHIS gathers data through personal interviews conducted in the respondent's household. The interviews are conducted by employees of the U.S. Census Bureau, following procedures specified by the NCHS. Currently, NHIS data are collected using a Computer-Assisted Personal Interviewer (CAPI) version of the NHIS questionnaire, in which the interviewer enters data directly into a laptop computer. Previously, data were collected using paper-and-pencil questionnaires.

The NHIS carries out sampling and data collection continuously throughout the year, using a multistage sampling plan:

1. 358 PSUs are selected from approximately 1900 available PSUs. The PSUs are geographic or governmental entities such as counties, groups of contiguous counties, or metropolitan statistical areas.
2. Samples of approximately four to twelve addresses are drawn from within each PSU, and all occupied households at the sample addresses are targeted for interview. Some information is collected on all members of the sampled households.
3. Within each targeted household, one adult and one child (if any) are selected for further interview.

The NHIS defines a household as an occupied housing unit, and a family as one person, or two or more related people living in the same household, or in some cases unrelated people such as an unmarried couple living in the same household. Each person within a household is described with a household reference number, according to their relationship to a household reference person, generally the person who owns or rents the housing unit. Respondents to the NHIS are also described by a family reference number, according to their relationship to the family reference person. In 98 percent of the households surveyed in the 2004 NHIS, the household consisted of one family so the family relationships and household relationships were identical. For the remaining 2 percent of cases, respondents have different family reference numbers and household reference numbers. Examples of this type of household include several unrelated roommates sharing living quarters, a family who rents part of their household to a renter and his or her child, and a family with a live-in housekeeper and his or her spouse.

The NHIS sample design was revised in 1995 and ensures that every state will be included in the NHIS. Although the NHIS data are insufficient to produce precise estimates at the state level, this sampling feature was included to facilitate the use of NHIS data with other state-level telephone surveys. Oversampling of African Americans and Hispanics was also included in the 1995 redesign, to allow more accurate estimates for those subgroups. In 2004, the NHIS collected data about 94,460 individuals in 37,466 families in 36,579 households, with a response rate of 86.9 percent.

Accessing Data and Ancillary Materials

NHIS data and ancillary materials are available in a variety of formats, depending on the year data were collected. Data for the years 1970 to 2002 are available in ASCII format on CD and may be purchased from the NCHS Data Dissemination Branch. Data for the years 1992 to 2004 are available for download from the NCHS website at http://www. cdc.gov/nchs/about/major/nhis/quest_data_related_doc.htm. Ancillary information available for each year's data includes documentation; questionnaires; flashcards; the Field Representative Manual and Survey Flowchart; Imputed Income Files; and SAS, SPSS, and Stata syntax files to convert the ASCII files and add variable formats. Questionnaires for the years 1962 to 1996 are available in the series "Current Estimates from the National Health Survey," published by the NCHS and available for download from the NHIS website cited previously. The NCHS created a Multiple Cause-of-Death data file that is available on CD-ROM and links NHIS respondents age 18 and older to the NDI. This data set allows researchers to conduct longitudinal and survival analysis that use death or cause of death as an outcome. NHIS respondents are included from the survey years 1986 to 1994, and NDI information is included through 1997. This CD-ROM may be ordered for free from the Information Dissemination Staff of the NCHS; it must be used in conjunction with the NHIS data file for the corresponding year.

The NHIS has constructed data files for the years 1993 and 1991 that allow the direct production of estimates of health factors at the state level. Statistical noise has been added to these data sets to protect confidentiality, while also allowing release of data with state identifiers. Small states were combined into groups to increase the sample size. These data files are available only in SAS format and are available, along with documentation, for purchase from the NTIS.

The Joint Canada/United States Survey of Health

The JCUSH is a one-time survey, conducted from 2002 to 2003, with a random sample of adults age 18 and older in Canada and the United States. JCUSH was conducted by Statistics Canada and the NCHS, and was the first survey to collect comprehensive information about health and health care access in both countries using a standard survey instrument and approach. Data collected by the JCUSH included demographic and socioeconomic factors, health status, health behaviors and risk factors, access to health care services, health care utilization including mental health and dentistry, and satisfaction with health care.

Focus

The JCUSH collected data that would allow national comparisons to be made between Canada and the United States in five areas: health status, risk factors, income differences and health, access to health care, and quality and satisfaction with health care. Information was collected in the following categories: household information; general health; activity limitation; chronic conditions; depression; mental health utilization; smoking; health status; height and weight; health care needs and utilization; medication use; mammography and Papanicolaou smear testing; dental visits; insurance; patient satisfaction; physical activity; sociodemographic characteristics, and income and wealth.

Data Collection

The JCUSH was administered to a stratified random sample of noninstitutionalized adults age 18 and older living in Canada or the United States at the time of the survey. Households were selected using random-digit-dial technology, and data were collected by regional offices of Statistics Canada using Computer-Assisted Telephone Interviewing (CATI). The sample was designed so reliable national estimates could be made for three age categories: 18 to 44 years, 45 to 64 years, and age 65 and older. Surveys were administered in English or Spanish in the United States and English or French in Canada. Response rates were 66 percent in Canada and 50 percent in the United States, and 3505 Canadians and 5183 Americans were included in the JCUSH.

Accessing Data and Ancillary Materials

The JCUSH data and ancillary data are available for download from the JCUSH website (http://www.cdc.gov/nchs/about/major/nhis/jcush_mainpage.htm). The data are in text format. Ancillary materials available from the website include the questionnaire in English, French, and Spanish; data set documentation; and SAS and SPSS code to translate the data and add formats.

The Longitudinal Studies of Aging

The LSOAs consist of four surveys studying two cohorts. These surveys were designed to study longitudinal changes in the health, functional status, living arrangements, and health services of older Americans as they age. The LSOAs is a collaborative effort of the National Institute on Aging and the NCHS. The LSOAs began in 1984, and data were most recently collected in 2000.

Focus

The LSOAs began with the 1984 *Supplement on Aging* (SOA), a study conducted by the NCHS as a supplement to the 1984 NHIS. The objectives of the SOA were to form the basis for a longitudinal study and to collect information on the health and social status of people age 55 years and older and on the interaction of health, psychosocial, and environmental factors in this population. The SOA also served as baseline data for the LSOA, which collected data over a 6-year period from individuals who were age 70 years and older at the time of their NHIS interview. The purposes of the LSOA included gathering information on the health status of older adults, measuring change in their functional status and living arrangements, measuring their health care utilization over time, and providing mortality rates broken down by demographic, social, economic, and health characteristics.

The SOA II replicates the SOA I about 10 years later, with a new cohort of people age 70 and older. SOA II closely resembles SOA I in methodology and content, and was conducted as a supplement to the 1994 NHIS on a random sample of civilian, noninstitutionalized persons included in the NHIS sample. It was conceived partly as a replication of the first SOA to determine if there had been changes in the level of disability of older persons between 1984 and 1994, and also served as the baseline for the LSOA II. Other goals of SOA II included gathering information about the correlates of changes in health and functioning of older Americans, the sequences of health events for this population, and the consequences of disability for them.

Data Collection

The SOA was conducted as a supplement to the 1984 NHIS, so data were collected in the same manner as the rest of the NHIS data, through personal interviews conducted in the respondent's home. The SOA sample was nationally representative of civilian, noninstitutionalized adults age 55 and older living in the United States, and data were collected from 16,148 individuals. The SOA data files include data from three sources. Information drawn from the 1984 NHIS includes demographics, activity restriction and limitation, bed-days, chronic and acute conditions, physician visits, and hospital stays. Information drawn from the 1984

Health Insurance Supplement includes health insurance coverage and type. Information collected from the 1984 SOA includes family structure, housing, relationships and social contacts, use of community services, income sources, health conditions and impairments, activities and instrumental activities of daily living, utilization of health services, and opinions on health matters.

The SOA served as the baseline for the first LSOA. The SOA cohort of 7527 adults age 70 years and older (not age 55 and older, as in the SOA) were followed for 6 years and were interviewed three more times, in 1986, 1988, and 1990. Follow-up interviews were conducted using CATI by U.S. Census Bureau employees. Records for LSOA participants were also linked to Medicare records, the NDI, and Multiple Cause-of-Death records. The LSOA data file therefore includes data from nine sources: the 1984 NHIS, 1984 Health Insurance Supplement, and 1984 SOA, as described previously; and the three 1986 to 1990 LSOA follow-up interviews, Medicare records, the NDI, and Multiple Cause-of-Death records. Data collected in the LSOA follow-up interviews include information on living arrangements, institutionalization, occupation, physical and activity limitations, nursing home and hospital stays, contacts with doctors, and economic information (1990 only). Data drawn from Medicare records include hospitalization, surgical procedures, home health care, hospice, and outpatient procedures. Data drawn from the NDI include date of death and certainty of match. Data drawn from Multiple Cause-of-Death records include underlying cause of death, up to eight causes of death, and whether an autopsy was performed.

SOA II was conducted as a supplement to the 1994 NHIS so data were collected through personal interviews conducted in the respondent's home, in the same manner as the rest of the NHIS data. The sample was nationally representative of civilian, noninstitutionalized adults age 70 and older living in the United States; data were collected from 9447 individuals. The SOA II data file includes information from four sources: the 1994 NHIS, the 1994 Family Resources Supplement to the NHIS, 1994 NHIS Survey on Disability, and SOA II. Data drawn from the 1994 NHIS include demographics, activity restriction and limitation, bed-days, chronic and acute conditions, physician visits, and hospital stays. Data drawn from the 1994 Family Resources Supplement include unmet needs for care and reasons for it. Data drawn from the 1994 NHIS Survey on Disability include mental health, substance abuse, mental health services, unmet needs for mental health services and the reason for them, unmet needs for other health services and the reasons those needs were unmet. Data gathered in SOA II include family structure and living arrangements, housing and long-term care, social relationships, physical functioning, chronic conditions, health opinions and behaviors, use of health, personal care and social services, use of assistive devices, health insurance, employment, and transportation.

The SOA II served as the baseline for LSOA II. The SOA II cohort of 9447 adults age 70 years and older were followed for 6 years and were interviewed two more times: from 1997 to 1998 and from 1999 to 2000. Follow-up interviews were conducting using CATI and were conducted by U.S. Census Bureau employees. In the future, records for LSOA participants will be linked to Medicare records, the NDI, and Multiple Cause-of-Death records. Data included currently in the LSOA II file are similar to those in LSOA I, with the exclusion of the linked records. Data are included from the 1994 NHIS, the 1994 Family Resources Supplement, the 1994 NHIS Survey on Disability, SOA II, and the LSOA II follow-up interviews of 1997 to 1998 and 1999 to 2000.

Accessing Data and Ancillary Materials

Data for SOA I and II and LSOA I and II are available on CD-ROM and may be requested from the CDC. Descriptions of the surveys and the data they contain, including questionnaires for the SOA I and II, are available from the appropriate section of the LSOAs website (http://www.cdc.gov/nchs/about/otheract/aging/soa1.htm) for the SOA I. Ancillary information available from the website includes descriptions of the surveys and data files, questionnaires, and links to reports about the surveys.

The State and Local Area Integrated Telephone Survey

The SLAITS is a set of data collection techniques developed by the NCHS, which is used to conduct a number of different health-related surveys at the national, state, and local levels. Each survey or module conducted using SLAITS has a sponsor, which may be a government agency, educational institution, or nonprofit organization. Each survey or module using SLAITS is developed to meet the needs of the survey sponsors. Topics covered in current and completed surveys include health insurance coverage, access to care, perceived health status, health care utilization, and child well-being and welfare.

Focus

The primary purpose of SLAITS is to provide efficient and timely methods to gather information needed to develop and implement programs and policies. SLAITS also allows the collection of data designed to provide statistically valid analyses at the state and local levels, even if the data are collected at a national level. SLAITS questionnaires are customized for each survey sponsor and may include standard questions drawn from other governmental surveys, as well as customized questions addressing particular state or local concerns. Some of the surveys were national and some were conducted in only a few states, depending on the needs of the sponsor. Six surveys or modules have been conducted or are currently being conducted using SLAITS: the *Health Module* (Iowa and Washington, 1997), the *Child Well-Being and Welfare Module* (Texas and Minnesota, 1998–1999), the *National Survey of Early Childhood Health* (national, 2000), the *National Survey of Children with Special Health Care Needs* (national, 2001 and 2005–2006), the *National Survey of Children's Health* (national, 2003–2004), and the *National Asthma Survey* (national, 2003–2004; Alabama, California, Illinois, and Texas, 2003–2004).

The Health Module was sponsored by the Office of the Assistant Secretary for Planning and Evaluation of the U.S. Department for Health and Human Services (DHHS). It drew questions from the NHIS and the Survey of Income and Program Participations, and was pilot-tested in Iowa (2675 persons, 1021 households) and Washington (2866 persons, 1068 households) in 1997. Data collected include family composition race/ethnicity; age; education; health care needs and utilization, including mental health and dentistry; health status and limitations; health insurance coverage and sources of payment; and employment and sources of income.

The Child Well-Being and Welfare Module was sponsored by the Office of the Assistant Secretary for Planning and Evaluation of DHHS. It used questions from various national surveys to investigate the association between participation in public assistance programs and factors believed to relate to child well-being, such as health care coverage, child care, safe neighborhoods, and parental employment. It was pilot-tested in 1998 and 1999 on a randomly selected sample of low-income families in Texas and a list sample of families receiving Medicaid or Minnesota Care (low-income health insurance) in Texas and Minnesota (2192 children total). Households with an income of less than 200 percent of the poverty level and with a child younger than 18 years of age were oversampled in Texas. Data collected include household composition, race/ethnicity, age, health insurance coverage, education, neighborhood safety and social climate, child behavior, amount and sources of family income, and employment.

The National Survey of Early Childhood Health was sponsored by the American Academy of Pediatrics, the Maternal and Child Health Bureau, and the American Academy of Pediatrics Friends of Children Fund. It was conducted in 2000 with a national sample of the parents of 2068 children: Hispanic and African American children, and children age 4 to 35 months, were oversampled. The survey's purpose was to provide national baseline data on pediatric care from the parent's point of view. Data collected include family composition, race/ethnicity, health care access and utilization, satisfaction with health care, child health and safety, parental receipt of medical information, parent–child interaction, child care, parental and child health, health insurance, and household income.

The National Survey of Children with Special Health Care Needs is sponsored by the Maternal and Child Health Bureau of the Health Resources and Services Administration (HRSA) and the Office of the Assistant Secretary for Planning and Evaluation of DHHS. It was conducted in all fifty states and the District of Columbia in 2001, and is being conducted again from 2005 to 2006. The survey assesses the prevalence and impact of children with special health care needs. More than 3000 households with children per state were screened to identify 750 (in 2001) or 850 (in 2005–2006) households having children with special needs.

Information collected includes race/ethnicity, health and functional status, health care needs and utilization, care coordination, satisfaction with care, health insurance and its adequacy, impact on the family, income, and Medicaid and State Children's Health Insurance Program (or S-CHIP) knowledge.

The National Survey of Children's Health was sponsored by the Maternal and Child Health Bureau of HRSA. It was conducted from 2003 to 2004 with a national sample of the parents of 102,353 children age 0 to 17 years. The focus was children's physical and emotional health and factors that may influence it, such as safe neighborhoods, school and afterschool experiences, family interactions, parental health, and medical care. Data collected include family composition, race/ethnicity, age, gender, languages spoken in the home, health and functional status, health insurance, health care access and utilization, satisfaction with health care, sports and social activities, parent–child interaction, family dynamics, parental health, neighborhood characteristics, employment, and income.

The National Asthma Survey was sponsored by the National Center for Environmental Health of the CDC. It was conducted from 2003 to 2004 with a national sample and also from 2003 to 2004 with a four-state sample (Alabama, California, Illinois, and Texas). The focus of the survey was the health care experiences of person with asthma, and health, socioeconomic, behavioral, and environmental factors that relate to the control of asthma. Data collected include age, gender, education, height and weight, income, asthma symptoms and history, health care utilization, activity limitations due to asthma, knowledge of asthma symptoms and care, household environment and modifications, employment and occupational exposure to chemicals, medication use, and family history of asthma.

Data Collection

SLAITS uses the same sampling frame and random-digit-dial telephone survey approach used by the NIS, and data are collected by the National Opinion Research Center under contract to NCHS. The survey design, sampling plan, and estimation procedures are different for each survey. Specific information is available from the relevant sections of the SLAITS website (http://www.cdc.gov/nchs/slaits.htm). Information about each survey is contained in a separate section within this website. For instance, information about the National Asthma Survey is available at http://www.cdc.gov/nchs/about/major/slaits/nas.htm.

Accessing Data and Ancillary Materials

Data collected through SLAITS is available in SAS format for download through the SLAITS website and can also be requested on CD-ROM from the NCHS. Ancillary information is also available from the SLAITS website, including questionnaires, methodologic information about each survey, bibliographies of papers and presentations using SLAITS data, frequency tables of responses to survey questions, and SAS code.

Fertility and Mortality Data

This chapter discusses seven sources of fertility and mortality data for the United States. Through the *National Vital Statistics System* (NVSS), the NCHS collects and makes available in one location information about vital events (births, deaths, marriages, divorces, and fetal deaths) in the United States and U.S. territories. The *Compressed Mortality File* (CMF) contains information about U.S. deaths in the years 1968 to 2002, aggregated to the county level and weighted to represent the national population for a given year. The *National Death Index* (NDI) is a centralized index of death record information within which the NCHS will perform searches to inform researchers of the vital status and cause of death of their subjects. The *National Mortality Followback Survey* (NMFS) collects information through interviews and administrative sources on a sample of individuals who died in the United States in a given year. It is conducted periodically, and each administration has focused on different topics, which have included risk factors, disability, health care utilization, and the reliability of death certificate information. The *National Maternal and Infant Health Survey* (NMIHS) was the first national survey to collect data on births, fetal deaths, and infant deaths simultaneously. It was conducted in 1988, with a Longitudinal Followup (LF) in 1991. The *Pregnancy Risk Assessment Monitoring System* (PRAMS) collects data that supplements that available on birth certificates, including maternal experiences and attitudes during pregnancy, while giving birth, and shortly after giving birth. It is an ongoing study that was initiated in 1987. The *National Survey of Family Growth* (NSFG) collects national data on marriage, divorce, contraception, infertility, and maternal and infant health; it has been conducted periodically since 1973, with the most recent administration in 2002.

The National Vital Statistics System

The NVSS is a cooperative enterprise in which information about vital events (births, deaths, marriages, divorces, and fetal deaths) is collected and disseminated by the NCHS from the jurisdictions legally responsible for maintaining registries of vital events and issuing copies of birth, marriage, divorce, and death certificates. The jurisdictions included in the NVSS are each of the fifty states, the District of Columbia, New York City, and the territories of Puerto Rico, the Virgin Islands, Guam, American Samoa, and the Commonwealth of the Northern Mariana Islands.

Focus

The NVSS natality data files contain information about births occurring in the United States; they do not include births to U.S. citizens living outside the United States. Information available in the current *Detail* files (records of individual births) includes residence of mother; age of father and mother; Apgar scores; birth weights; gender of child; education of father and mother; gestational period; race and ethnicity of father, mother, and child; parents' marital status; time since last birth, fetal death, or pregnancy termination; mother's place of birth; prenatal care; and attendant at birth.

The NVSS mortality data files include information about deaths occurring in the United States; they do not contain information about the deaths of U.S. citizens who died outside the United States. There are two main types of mortality data files: *Underlying Cause-of-Death* and *Multiple Cause-of-Death*. The principal difference between the two types of files is that the Underlying Cause-of-Death file includes only one cause of death, while the Multiple Cause-of-Death file may include more than one cause. Data collected in the current Detail files (records of individual deaths) include residence of decedent, age at death, gender, education, race and ethnicity, employment, place of birth and death, marital status, manner of death, and cause(s) of death.

The NVSS fetal death files contain information about all fetal deaths (death of a fetus before complete expulsion or extraction from the mother) occurring in the United States. Data available vary by state but may include mother's residence; mother's and father's age; mother's alcohol and tobacco use; birth weight; attendant at delivery; mother's and father's education; gestational period; mother's and father's race and ethnicity; child's race and gender; medical risk factors; mother's pregnancy history, including weight gain during pregnancy; medical risk factors; and complications of labor or delivery.

The *Linked Birth and Infant Death* files contain information drawn from the birth certificates and death certificates of infants who died at younger than 1 year of age in the United States, Puerto Rico, the Virgin Islands, and Guam. Data available in these files include age; race and ethnicity of the mother and father; birth weight and gestational age; plurality (whether the child was a singleton, twin, triplet, etc.); prenatal care history; mother's education; marital status; maternal smoking; age at death; and underlying and multiple causes of death.

Marriage and divorce data are collected from certificates of marriage and divorce for states that meet reporting criteria (discussed in more detail later). Data in the marriage files differ by state and year of collection but may include date of marriage, type of ceremony, and bride and groom's age, as well as education, number of marriages, previous marital status, time since previous marriage, race, state of birth, and state of residence. Divorce file data also vary by year and state but may include date of marriage, date of separation, duration of marriage, number of children younger than 18 years, total number of children, custody of children, state of divorce, husband and wife's age at marriage and separation, education, number of marriages, race, state of marriage, and state of residence.

Data Collection

The public-use natality data files contain information drawn from birth certificates. For the years 1968 to 1971, the natality files included a 50 percent sample of births; since 1972, they have included all births occurring in all states participating in the Vital Statistics Cooperative Program (VSCP). In 1972, six states participated in the VSCP; since 1985, all states and the District of Columbia have participated. For the years 1969 to 1988, natality data are available in three formats: *Detail, State summary,* and *Local summary.* Detail files are formatted so one record in the file corresponds to one birth, and includes detailed information on the mother, father, and birth. State summary and Local summary files include fewer data fields, and are aggregated at the state or local level and weighted to represent the total number of births in a given state or local area. They include birth weight plus demographic information such as race and gender of the child and age of the mother. Natality Detail files are also available for the years 1989 to 2000.

The public-use mortality files contain data drawn from death certificates. For the years 1968 to 1971, 1973 to 1980, and 1983 to 2002, information was included for all death certificates. In 1972, data were collected from a 50 percent sample of death certificates. In 1981 and 1982, data for the multiple cause files were drawn from a 50 percent sample of nineteen registration areas, while the underlying cause files for those years were based on all death certificates for those years. Detail mortality files are currently available for the years 1968 to 2002, and Local Area summary files for the year 1968 to 1988. The meanings of detail and summary files are the same as for natality data.

The public-use fetal death files contain information collected from fetal death certificates. Data from these files are not completely comparable across states because of differences in state laws. Some states require that all fetal deaths be reported, while others only require reporting of gestations of 20 weeks or longer. Data are available for the United States for the years 1982 to 1995; for 1994 and 1995, separate data sets are available for Puerto Rico, the Virgin Islands, and Guam. Fetal death information for the years 1995 to 1999 is also available in the *Perinatal Mortality Data Set*, which includes information on births, infant deaths, and fetal deaths for those years.

The Linked Birth and Infant Death files were created by the NCHS by combining information drawn from both the birth certificate and the death certificate of children who died at younger than 1 year of age. Linked Birth and Infant Death files are currently available for the years 1983 to 1991 and 1995 to 2002; they were not produced in 1992 to 1994. Two formats have been used to create these files, the *birth cohort format* and the *period format*. The two formats use the same denominator, which is all births occurring in a given year. However, the numerators differ. In the birth cohort format, the numerator is defined by the birth year so that for the 1991 file the numerator would be deaths to children born in 1991, whether the death occurred in 1991 or 1992. In the period format, the numerator is defined by the year of death, so the numerator for 1995 would include all infant deaths that occurred in that year, whether the child was born in 1994 or 1995. The birth cohort format was used exclusively in the years 1983 to 1991, while beginning in 1995, the Linked Birth and Infant Death files have been produced using both the birth cohort and the period format.

Public-use marriage data are drawn from certificates of marriage from states that are in the marriage registration area, meaning that they meet NVSS reporting criteria. In 1968 to 1970, thirty-nine states and the District of Columbia were included in the marriage registration area; by 1995, forty-one states and the District of Columbia were included. Records of each included state are sampled weighted to represent the total number of marriages in the state in question. Public-use marriage data are available for the years 1968 to 1990.

Public-use divorce data are drawn from certificates of divorce from states that are in the divorce registration area, meaning that they meet NVSS reporting criteria. In 1968, the divorce registration area included twenty-six states; in 1986 to 1990, it included thirty-one states and the District of Columbia. As with public-use marriage data, records of each included state are sampled and weighted to represent the total number of divorces in the state in question. Public-use divorce data are available for the years 1968 to 1990.

Accessing Data and Ancillary Materials

Public-use data files produced by the NVSS are available as ASCII files for purchase on CD-ROM from the NTIS or GPO and/or as data tapes from the NCHS. Detailed information on ordering is available from the "Publications and Information Products" page of the NCHS website (http://www.cdc.gov/nchs/products.htm). Researchers may apply to the Director of Vital Statistics for the creation of customized data files that include information such as exact dates of birth or death or identification of all counties. If the request is approved, the customized file may be released to the researcher, or the researcher may be required to access it at the NCHS RDC.

Standard forms, substantially revised in 2003, and model procedures for the registration of vital events have been developed cooperatively by the NCHS and the responsible jurisdictions. Copies of the forms and explanations of the procedures are available from the NVSS website (http://www.cdc.gov/nchs/nvss.htm).

The NVSS does not issue copies of birth, death, marriage, or divorce certificates, which must be requested from the appropriate jurisdiction. Links to the offices that handle these requests are available from the NCHS website (http://www.cdc.gov/nchs/howto/w2w/w2welcom.htm). In addition, more recent or detailed information regarding vital statistics in a particular jurisdiction may be available from these local offices.

The Compressed Mortality File

The CMF is based on NCHS data about deaths in the United States for the years 1968 to 2002, aggregated to the county level and weighted to represent the national population for a given year. It permits calculation of death rates and trends at the national and subnational levels, and permits further breakdown by age, race, and gender.

Focus

The CMF consists of a reduced set of information about deaths that occurred in the United States in the years 1968 to 2002, aggregated to the county level and weighted to allow national and subnational estimates. This file was created to allow many years of data to be included in a single file, to allay concerns about confidentiality, and to allow researchers to study death rates and trends across the United States with breakdowns by a few major demographic variables.

Data Collection

The CMF consists of two files: a mortality file and a population file. The CMF mortality file is based on NCHS mortality files, in which the unit of analysis is an individual death. Data for the year 1972 are based on a 50 percent sample of deaths, each of which is weighted by 2; for each subsequent year, the CMF is based on the entire population of deaths for the year. The following data are included in the CMF: state and county of residence, year of death (not the full date), race (White, Black, or other), gender, age group (sixteen categories) at death, underlying cause of death (four-digit ICD code), and recoded cause of death (to allow for change in ICD codes over the years 1968–2002). Data are aggregated on all data fields, and a count variable is added to indicate the number of identical records. The CMF population file is based on U.S. Bureau of the Census estimates of the population of the United States, each state, and each county.

Accessing Data and Ancillary Materials

CMF data for the years 1968 to 1988 are contained in a single public-use file that may be purchased on CD-ROM from the NTIS or on data tape from the NCHS. Because of confidentiality concerns, access to data for the years 1989 to 1998 and 1999 to 2002 must be requested from NCHS, including an explanation of how the data will be used and how confidentiality will be maintained.

It is possible to access CMF data through a menu-based interface on the CDC Wonder website, which allows calculation of the number of deaths, crude and age-adjusted death rates by residence (county, state, or entire United States), age group, race, gender, year of death, and underlying cause of death, for the years 1979 to 2002. Separate interfaces must be used for the years 1979 to 1998 and 1999 to 2002. The interfaces may be accessed from http://wonder.cdc.gov/mortArchives.html and detailed information about technical issues (e.g., how the U.S. population figures were estimated in different years) is available at http://wonder.cdc.gov/wonder/help/mort.html.

The National Death Index

The NDI is a centralized index of death record information established by the NCHS to allow researchers to discover or confirm the vital status of their subjects. Researchers do not have direct access to NDI information but can submit a proposal to the NDI explaining why they want a search of the NDI performed. If their proposal is approved, researchers then submit data about persons for whom they want the NDI to be searched, and the NDI staff returns a report that indicates possible matches for each person searched, including state of death, death certificate, and date of death. *NDI Plus* is an expanded service that also supplies cause of death codes for the better matches.

Focus

The NDI allows researchers to determine the vital status of individuals in a single step rather than having to request searches in each state in which a person might have died. If NDI finds one or more matches for an individual, the researcher can then use the information provided to request death certificates from the state in question to determine which match, if any, applies to the individual from their study, and to obtain further information such as cause(s) of death. Use of the NDI for legal, administrative, or genealogy purposes is expressly prohibited.

Data Collection

NDI information is collected from death records information on file in each state's vital statistics office. It is subject to the same limitations as death certificate information. For instance, if a U.S. citizen died outside the United States, he or she would not have a state death certificate and therefore would not be listed in the NDI. The NDI is updated about 12 months after the end of a year, using computer files submitted by state vital statistics offices. NDI data are currently available for the years 1979 to 2004.

Accessing Data and Ancillary Materials

Individual researchers do not have direct access to NDI data. Instead, the researcher must submit an application stating why he or she wants a search of NDI records to be performed. This proposal is considered by a twelve-person board similar to an Institutional Review Board; if it is approved, the researcher can then submit a list of persons for whom he or she wants an NDI search to be performed. Data about persons to be searched must be submitted in an electronic file in the format specified by the NDI. The exact specifications for submitting this data, plus other information such as explanations of NDI charges, NDI matching criteria, a sample retrieval report, and a downloadable application, are available on the NDI website (http://www.cdc.gov/nchs/ndi.htm).

The cost for NDI searches is based on the number of years searched, the number of individuals searched, whether the person's vital status is known or unknown, and whether cause of death codes will be included in the report. NDI searches combine information from a number of variables, and users are encouraged to submit as much of the following information as possible about each person they want to be searched: first and last name, middle initial, father's surname, social security number, exact day of birth, race, gender, marital status, state of birth, and state of residence. The NDI retrieval program recognizes seven combinations of criteria that qualify as a match, such as social security number alone; day and month of birth plus first and last name; and first and last name, month of birth, and year of birth within 1 year. The retrieval report indicates which criteria matched exactly, as well as the state and date of death and death certificate number. This information may be used by the researcher to choose which of multiple matches are most likely to refer to the individual sought, and may be used to request a death certificate from the state where the death occurred.

The National Mortality Followback Survey

The NMFS has been conducted periodically by the NCHS since 1961. Each NMFS draws a sample of individuals who died in the United States in a given year and supplements the death certificate information with information drawn from a variety of sources, including administrative data and an interview conducted with a proxy respondent, usually the decedent's next of kin or another person familiar with the decedent's life history. Each NMFS has focused on different issues: the most recent, conducted in 1993, collected data on socioeconomic factors, risk behaviors, disability, health care utilization, and reliability of death certificate information.

Focus

The NMFS gathers information, beyond that contained in the death certificate, on a representative sample of individuals who died in the United States in a given year. The first NMFS was conducted in 1961 and focused on hospital and institutional care in the last year of life. The 1962 to 1963 survey focused on socioeconomic differentials in mortality. The 1964 to 1965 survey included information on health insurance coverage, health care expenditures, and sources of payment for health care in the last year of life. The 1966 to 1968 survey focused on smoking and cancer mortality.

The 1986 NMFS focused on socioeconomic status, risk factors, and health care sought and provided in the last year of life. Data were gathered from three principal sources: (1) the death certificate; (2) an interview (primarily by mail, with telephone and/or in-person follow-up, if necessary) with a proxy respondent, preferably a relative familiar with the decedent's life history; and (3) a mailed questionnaire sent to the administrators of any health care institutions where the decedent spent at least one night in his or her last year of life. If no relative could be located to perform the interview and the decedent died in a nursing home, a shortened interview was conducted with a staff member who was familiar with the decedent.

Data gathered from the proxy interview includes education; income; medical history; activities of daily living; care used and source of payment, costs, and problems in getting care; exercise, alcohol, and smoking history; medicines used; social support; type of employment; spouse's occupational history; marital history; and family medical history. Data gathered from the facility questionnaire include dates of admissions and discharges; diagnoses; surgical and diagnostic procedures for each admission; and type of facility.

The 1993 NMFS focused on socioeconomic factors, risk factors, and health care services used in the last year of life, and disability in the last year of life. It gathered information from three sources: (1) death certificates; (2) an interview with a proxy respondent, as in the 1986 NMFS; and (3) data from the medical examiner/coroner abstract record for people who died because of accidental injury, homicide, or suicide.

Much of the data gathered in the 1993 proxy interview were similar to those collected in 1986, with the addition of questions about firearms, comorbid conditions, cognitive functioning, assistive and medical devices used, motor vehicle use, organ donorship, participation in social activities, life events, and problem behaviors. Data collected from the medical examiner/coroner abstract file included place of death, manner of death, firearm-related injury, circumstances of injury, autopsy, toxicologic findings, comorbid conditions, activities and impairments, medical devices implanted, and organ donorship.

Data Collection

The 1986 and 1993 NMFS both drew samples of death certificates from the *Current Mortality Sample* (CMS) for the relevant year. The CMS is a systematic 10 percent sample of death certificates as received by the NCHS from the individual states. The 1986 NMFS is a nationally representative sample of adults age 25 and older who died in 1986 and includes records from 18,773 deaths. All states except Oregon were included in the sample, and New York City and the District of Columbia were included as independent vital registration areas. Oregon did not participate because of the state's respondent consent requirements. The 1993 NMFS is a nationally representative sample of persons age 15 and older and includes records from 22,957 deaths. All states but South Dakota, plus New York City and the District of Columbia, were included in the 1993 NMFS. South Dakota did no participate because of a state law restricting the use of death certificate information for follow-back surveys. The 1993 NMFS includes oversampling of persons younger than age 35, African Americans, and women.

Accessing Data and Ancillary Materials

Data from the 1986 and 1993 NMFS in ASCII format are available for purchase on CD-ROM or data tapes from the NTIS. Ancillary materials, although not the data, for the 1993 NMFS may be downloaded from the NMFS website (http://www.cdc.gov/nchs/about/major/nmfs/nmfs.htm). Materials available include the questionnaires; information about the survey, data preparation and processing, and sample weights; and SAS and SUDAAN syntax, variable lists, and file format and response frequencies. The NMFS website also maintains links to research reports and a bibliography of articles using the NMFS.

The National Maternal and Infant Health Survey and Longitudinal Followup

The NMIHS was conducted in 1988, with an LF in 1991. It was the first national survey to collect data on births, fetal deaths, and infant deaths simultaneously, and it gathered data on demographic characteristics and socioeconomic status of mothers, prenatal care, pregnancy history, occupational background of mother, type and sources of medical care, and health status of mother and infant.

Focus

The NMIHS was conducted to gather more information than was available in vital records (birth, death, and fetal death certificates), with the primary objective of facilitating the study of factors related to poor pregnancy outcomes, including low birth weight, stillbirth, and infant illness and death. It was a follow-back study, meaning that the starting point was vital records (e.g., birth certificates) and that information was gathered from informants who were located or "followed back" from those records. The LF was conducted in 1991 to provide longitudinal information for a sample of the birth cohort interviewed for the NMIHS in 1988.

Data Collection

NMIHS data were collected by questionnaires mailed to a sample of mothers who gave birth or had a fetal or infant death in 1988; the samples are weighted to be representative of all births, fetal deaths, and infant deaths for 1988. Women were asked for permission to contact their health care providers. About 93 percent granted this, and additional information collected from questionnaires sent to these providers was added to the mother's file. Data were also drawn from the birth certificate, fetal death certificate, or infant death certificate. The NMIHS includes 9953 women who had live births (and whose infant did not die), 3309 who had fetal deaths, and 5332 who had infant deaths.

The mother's questionnaire was thirty-five pages long and includes detailed questions on prenatal care; mother's use of tobacco, alcohol, and drugs; use of birth control; breastfeeding; desire for the pregnancy; height and weight of mother and father; pregnancy history; marital history; education and employment of mother and father; race and national original of mother and father; health during pregnancy; infant health and use of health care; and child care. Data collected from health care providers include diagnostic and other procedures, medications, prenatal and postpartum care, infant health status and care, and diagnoses for baby's and mother's hospitalization.

The LF contains three parts: a survey of women who gave birth to live infants in 1988, a survey of women who had a fetal or infant death in 1988, and a survey of child medical providers. The live birth survey was conducted with all women who were interviewed for the 1988 live birth cohort. The response rate was 89 percent, yielding 8285 completed interviews. The fetal death and infant death survey was conducted with a subsample of women from the fetal death and infant death cohorts of the NMIHS. The response rate was 82 percent. The child medical provider survey was conducted with medical providers and hospitals named by participating women as those who diagnosed, treated, or admitted their child. The response rate was 89 percent for hospitals and 74 percent for pediatric care providers.

Data collected in the LF live birth survey included household composition; behavioral problems; injuries and illnesses; immunizations; medication use; safety information, such as car seat and smoke detector use; child care; maternal health; employment and receipt of public assistance; and health insurance. Data collected in the fetal and infant death survey questionnaire included counseling; subsequent pregnancies, adoptions, and foster care; maternal health; family employment, income, and receipt of public assistance; HIV testing; and maternal depression. Data collected in the LF medical provider survey included child's health; use of medical devices; immunizations; medications; pediatric visits and hospitalizations; and lab tests, including HIV testing.

Accessing Data and Ancillary Materials

Data for the NMIHS and LF are available for purchase on separate CD-ROMs from NCHS. Further information is available on the NCHS website at http://www.cdc.gov/nchs/products/elec_prods/subject/lfnmihs. htm#avail. Both CDs include documentation that provides a description of the survey, response rates, sample design, estimation procedures, methodologic notes, and weighting information. However, because of confidentiality concerns, the two files may not be merged except at the NCHS RDC.

The Pregnancy Risk Assessment Monitoring System

The PRAMS was initiated in 1987 with the goal of reducing adverse birth outcomes and improving the health of mothers and infants. This system collects data that supplement that available on birth certificates, and includes maternal experiences and attitudes during pregnancy, while giving birth, and shortly after giving birth. It is conducted cooperatively by the CDC and state health departments. Twenty-nine states plus New York City currently participate in PRAMS, and six other states have participated in the past.

Focus

The PRAMS was initiated in 1987 out of a concern that birth outcomes in the United States were not improving as expected. In particular, there was concern that the incidence of low-birth-weight infants was similar to what it had been 20 years previous and that infant mortality rates were not declining as sharply as they had in previous years. PRAMS data are collected at the state level because responsibility for programs to improve birth outcomes rests primarily with individual state health departments, and the data collected differs somewhat between states. However, some types of data are collected in all participating states, allowing comparisons among states.

Data Collection

PRAMS data are collected each month from a stratified sample of women in each state who recently gave birth to a live infant. Most data are collected by a questionnaire mailed to selected women 2 to 4 months after delivery. If they do not respond to repeated mailings, an interview will be conducted by telephone. Many states oversample low-birth-weight births, as well as race and ethnicity. Sampling weights are applied so the sample represents the entire population of births in the state.

The PRAMS questionnaire for each state is unique. It consists of two parts: *core* questions asked in all states (currently, sixty questions), and *standard questions* (currently, ten to twenty-six per state) that are either developed by the state in question or chosen by the state from a list of pretested questions supplied by the CDC. Topics included in core questions are attitudes and feelings about the pregnancy; content and source of prenatal care; use of alcohol and tobacco; physical abuse; pregnancy-related illness; infant health care; contraceptive use; and knowledge of pregnancy-related health issues, such as the benefits of folic acid and risks of HIV. Standard questions cover many topics: those available in 2004 include breastfeeding, living arrangements, and physical activity. PRAMS questionnaires are currently available in English and Spanish.

The PRAMS also includes data drawn from birth certificates, including maternal demographics and pregnancy outcomes. Information that could identify a particular birth, such as the birth certificate number and the infant's and mother's date of birth, are omitted from the PRAMS files.

Accessing Data and Ancillary Materials

Researchers who want to use PRAMS data from only one state should contact that state's PRAMS coordinator. Contact information for these individuals is available on the PRAMS website (http://www.cdc. gov/prams). Access to PRAMS data for multiple states must be requested from the CDC. The researcher must submit a proposal using the guidelines available on the PRAMS website, which will be reviewed by the CDC. Oral presentations and papers using PRAMS data must be submitted to the CDC and the states whose data are being used for approval. PRAMS questionnaires for the years 1995 to 2007 are available for download from the PRAMS website.

The National Survey of Family Growth

The NSFG has been conducted periodically since 1973 for the purpose of collecting national data on marriage, divorce, contraception, infertility, and maternal and infant health in the United States. The first five NSFG cycles were conducted in 1973, 1976, 1982, 1988, and 1995, and they collected information from women only. The most recent NSFG was conducted in 2002 and collected information from both men and women.

Focus

The original purpose of the NSFG was to collect nationally representative data on issues of fertility, marriage, and maternal and infant health. For the first five cycles (1973–1995), data were collected only from women age 15 to 44, thus including women in the age range most likely to give birth. For the 2002 cycle, data were also collected from men and included more detailed questions about sexual behavior than previous surveys.

Data Collection

Data for the first five NSFG cycles were obtained through personal interviews conducted in the respondents' homes. The survey sample was drawn from the civilian, noninstitutionalized population of women age 15 to 44 years in the United States. Each sample included about 8000 to 10,000 women. In cycles 1 to 3, only the 48 contiguous states were included in the survey; in cycles 4 to 5, Alaska and Hawaii were included. The 2002 NSFG was conducted with an area probability sample of the household population (both males and females) of the United States, age 15 to 44 years, and was also collected through in-person home interviews. For the 2002 NSFG, 7643 women and 4928 men were interviewed.

Data for the first five NSFG cycles is collected into two types of files: a *respondent* file and an *interval* or *pregnancy* file. NSFG questions have varied over the years, but the respondent file has always contained information about the woman interviewed. Over the years, the respondent file has included information such as living arrangements; work and education history; number of pregnancies, adoption, and other children raised; marriage and cohabitation history; use of contraception; demographic characteristics, including race, religion, and income; health insurance; income; and child care. The interval or pregnancy file has always contained information about topics such as pregnancies, prenatal care, contraceptive use, and births.

Data for the 2002 NSFG was collected into three types of files: a *female respondent* file, a *male respondent* file, and a *female pregnancy* file. Data collected in the female respondent file include demographic information about the woman; pregnancies and adoptions; marriages and cohabitations; use of contraceptives, family planning services, and sterilizations; infertility; attitudes toward pregnancy; and health insurance. The male respondent file includes data on similar topics, except for the pregnancy information. The female pregnancy file contains detailed pregnancy histories for the woman, including whether a pregnancy was planned, and selected respondent characteristics.

Certain data collected in the NSFG are not publicly available but can be made available to researchers through special application to the NSFG. This applies to three types of data: sensitive information collected through Audio Computer-Assisted Self-Interviewing (ACASI), interviewer variables, and contextual data. ACASI was used to collect information on topics such as pregnancy terminations, condom use, sexual orientation, types of sexual activity, and number of sexual partners. ACASI data and documentation are available from NSFG free of charge to researchers who supply a description of their proposed use of the data and who sign a User Agreement (available from the NSFG website). Interviewer data are available through application to the NCHS RDC. Further information is available from the RDC website (http://www.cdc.gov/nchs/r&d/rdc.htm). Contextual data, which describe the social geographic context for each respondent, are available for the NSFG through application to the NCHS RDC. Contextual data for the 2002 NSFG are drawn from four sources: the 2000 U.S. Census, the County and City Data Book, a county-level file of family planning services, and a county-level file of sexually transmitted disease information. Researchers may also request that other contextual variables be added to existing NSFG data files.

NSFG data collection procedures are designed to permit analysis at the national level, at the level of the four major Census regions (Northeast, Midwest, South, and West) and for metropolitan versus nonmetropolitan areas. State-level analysis is not supported.

Accessing Data and Ancillary Materials

NSFG data files for the first five cycles are available free on CD-ROM from the NCHS. Each CD-ROM contains documentation, including an explanation of file organization, how missing data were imputed, how dates are coded, a summary of sample design and variance estimation issues, and a codebook. NSFG data are also available on data tapes that may be purchased from the NTIS. The NSFG questionnaires may be downloaded from the NSFG website at http://www.cdc.gov/nchs/nsfg.htm. The NSFG website also includes a bibliography of publications using the NSFG, as well as links to press releases and federal reports based on the NSFG.

Medicare and Medicaid Data

Medicare and Medicaid are U.S. governmental health insurance programs administered by the Centers for Medicare and Medicaid Services (CMS), formerly known as the Health Care Financing Administration. Both programs were signed into law on July 30, 1965, by President Lyndon B. Johnson. Medicare is a federal health insurance program for people age 65 and older, people with certain disabilities, and people with end-stage renal disease (ESRD), and has two principal parts (not including the prescription drug element begun in 2006). Medicare Part A is hospital insurance, which most Americans automatically become eligible for on their sixty-fifth birthday. Coverage under Part A does not require the payment of premiums, although there are deductible and coinsurance payments. Medicare Part B is optional medical insurance, primarily for outpatient care and doctor's services, and requires payment of monthly premiums. However, 95 percent of those eligible for Part B choose to participate. Medicaid is a state-administered health insurance program, primarily for people who are low income and for those with disabilities, that is partially financed by the federal government. Eligibility and benefits for Medicaid differ by state.

Most of the data sets discussed in this chapter contain primarily administrative data, most often evidence of medical claims paid by either the Medicaid or the Medicare system. Particularly in the case of Medicaid, therefore, researchers must be cautious about interpreting data in these files as representing the total health care needs or utilization of persons enrolled in either system because evidence of any care not paid for through the Medicaid or Medicare system would not be included in these data. Two surveys are also discussed: the *Medicare Current Beneficiary Study* (MCBS) and the *Medicare Health Outcomes Study* (HOS).

CMS classifies data files into three categories, depending on the level of personal information available in each. More restrictions apply to files in which individual people are identified by a specific variable, such as social security number or Unique Physician Identification Number, or could be identified by a combination of variables such as date of birth, race, gender, and ZIP code. The highest level of restrictions applies to *Research Identifiable Files* (RIFs), which include specific identifiers such as beneficiary social security numbers. Researchers who want to use RIFs must submit a formal request to the Research Data Assistance Center (ResDAC; go to http://www.resdac.umn.edu or send an e-mail to resdac@umn.edu), including a Data User Agreement and study plan or protocol. In addition, users must pay processing costs, which can add up to thousands of dollars. A lower level of restrictions applies to *Beneficiary Encrypted Files* (BEFs), also known as *Limited Data Set* files, in which personal identifiers have been encrypted or blanked out. It is also necessary to apply to the ResDAC for access to BEFs, and costs are similar to that for RIFs; however, it is easier to get permission to use BEFs. The lowest level of restrictions applies to *Public Use Files* (PUFs), which are generally aggregated to levels higher than the individual (i.e., to the state level) and contain no beneficiary-level or physician-level information. Some information in the PUFs is summarized from RIFs, and some is available only through the PUFs. Information about ordering the PUFs, which are much cheaper than BEFs and RIFs, is available on the CMS website (http://www.cms.hhs.gov/NonIdentifiableDataFiles/).

The major types of Medicare files, available as either RIFs or BEFs, are

- The *Denominator Record* files, which contain basic demographic and enrollment information about persons enrolled in and/or entitled to Medicare in a given year
- *Standard Analytical Files* (SAFs), which contain information about Medicare claims, for both Part A and Part B; each SAF record represents a final action claim, after algorithms have resolved any adjustments
- *Medicare Provider Analysis and Review* (MedPAR) files, which contain information about stays in inpatient hospitals and skilled nursing facilities (SNFs); each MedPAR record represents a stay in an inpatient

hospital or SNF, including all services rendered from time of admission to discharge, and may represent one or several claims
• *Prospective Payment System* (PPS) files, which contain claims-level data from the hospital Outpatient Prospective Payment System (OPPS) and Partial Hospitalization Programs (PHPs)

Many RIFs and BEFs are available as both 100 percent and 5 percent files. The 100 percent files include all records for a given time period, while the 5 percent files contain a 5 percent systematic sample of records (those with the values 05, 20, 45, 70, or 95 in positions 8 and 9 of the Health Insurance Claim number).

The Medicare Denominator Record Files

The Medicare Denominator Files contain a record for each person enrolled in and/or entitled to Medicare Part A, Part B, or both, in a given year. Denominator files are available as RIFs for the years 1991–2004; as BEFs, they are available for the years 1999–2005, as either a 100 percent file (all records), or a 5 percent sample. RIF Denominator Files are available from CMS on tape cartridges. The BEF 5 percent denominator file is available on CD-ROM from CMS and the 100 percent file is available on DVD. Record layouts for all three types of denominator file are available on the "Identifiable Files" section of the CMS webpage, as is COBOL and SAS code for the BEFs (http://www.cms.hhs.gov/IdentifiableDataFiles/01_Overview.asp#TopOfPage), as is COBOL and SAS code for the BEFs. All three types of Denominator Record Files become available in May of the year following that of the data collected (e.g., 2000 data becomes available in May 2001).

Data available in Medicare Denominator Record Files include relationship of beneficiary to primary beneficiary (i.e., if a wife qualified as a beneficiary through her husband); state, county, and ZIP code of residence; date of birth; gender; race/ethnicity; age at end of prior year; original and current reasons for entitlement; ESRD status; Medicare status; reason for termination of Part A (including death); reason for termination of Part B; Entitlement/Buy-in; health maintenance organization membership; months of coverage for Part A and Part B; date of death; and reference year of enrollment.

The Standard Analytical Files

There are seven categories of Medicare SAFs, each of which contains one type of claim. The types of SAFs are Physician/Supplier, Outpatient, Inpatient, Home Health Agency, Hospice, Skilled Nursing Facility, and Durable Medical Equipment. In most cases (if it would not violate confidentiality), SAF data are available as either a 100 percent or 5 percent sample. Record layouts for SAFs are available in the "Identifiable Data Files" page of the CMS website cited previously. In addition, SAS and COBOL syntax and data element lists are available for the BEF files. RIFs are available for the years 1991 to 2004 on tape cartridge; BEFs are available on CD, DVD, or hard drive.

The specific information included in an SAF varies somewhat according to the type of claim contained in the file. However, all SAFs are based on claims data and typically include information such as beneficiary demographic data (race, gender, date of birth, state and county of residence), diagnosis (ICD-9 code), and amount of claim.

The Medicare Provider Analysis and Review Files

The MedPAR files were developed to facilitate the study of inpatient hospital and SNF care. Each hospital or SNF stay is represented in a MedPAR file by a single record that contains ICD-9 diagnosis and procedure codes, procedure dates, and diagnosis-related group (DRG). A MedPAR record may represent one or more claims because it contains information about all services rendered from time of admission to discharge for a single beneficiary. About 90 percent of inpatient stays and 50 percent of SNF stays involve a single claim. Since 1999, claims from managed care organizations have been excluded.

MedPAR files contain claims data for services provided to Medicare beneficiaries admitted to Medicare-certified inpatient hospitals and SNFs. Information available includes beneficiary demographic and entitlement data, diagnosis and surgery information, use of hospital or SNF resources, days of care, and detailed charge data. Date of death information is appended to a MedPAR record if it occurs within 3 years of date of discharge. RIFs are available on data cartridge for the calendar or fiscal years 1991 to 2003; the 2002 MedPAR file alone contains more than 12 million records. The MedPAR BEF data are kept in three separate files: one for inpatient hospital data, one for SNF data, and one for long-term care hospital (LTCH) data. Although data identifying individuals have been removed or encrypted from BEFs, hospitals, SNFs, and LTCHs are identified by their six-digit Medicare billing number.

The Prospective Payment System Files

The Medicare PPS was introduced in 1983 as a means to encourage cost-efficient management of medical care by changing the financial incentives offered to hospitals. In the PPS, patients are classified into DRGs, and hospitals are paid a predetermined amount for each patient admitted in a particular DRG, regardless of services provided by the hospital. The PPS was first applied to hospitals and was expanded to SNFs in 1997 and to outpatient care in 2000. Outpatient care reimbursements are based on Ambulatory Payment Classifications (APCs), which are comparable to DRGs; more than 660 APCs have currently been defined. SNFs are reimbursed through a per diem system, where they receive a fixed rate of reimbursement for each day of care for each patient, adjusted for case mix and geographic variation in wages.

Patients are classified into DRGs using information that appears on the patient's medical record, including age, gender, principal diagnosis, complications and comorbidities (CCs), surgical procedures, and discharge disposition. DRG categories are design by CMS to be "clinically coherent," meaning that patients in a similar DRG should have a similar clinical condition. Examples of common DRGs are "Heart Failure and Shock," "Simple Pneumonia & Pleurisy Age >17 with CC," and "Specific Cerebrovascular Disorders except TIA." PPS payments are based on the average cost for treating patients in a given DRG. Exception is made for patients with very high costs, known as "outliers."

PPS data are available as RIFs or BEFs. The hospital OPPS RIF file is a claims-level file and includes information from 2004 hospital outpatient

PPS claims that were paid by June 2005. It is available on cartridge and contains more than 58 million records. OPPS data include provider, dates of care, bill type, diagnosis codes, outlier indication, services, charges, costs, and payments. A separate RIF contains information about claims from the PHP, which refers to day treatment programs in which the beneficiary does not stay overnight in the treatment facility. The PHP file for 2004 includes more than 154,000 claims from hospitals and community mental health centers and is available on cartridge. This file contains claims from the same time period as the OPPS 2004 file, and the records contain similar information.

BEF PPS files are available for the same time period as the RIF files and can be purchased on DVD. There are three BEF files containing PPS information. The OPPS and PHP files correspond to the RIF versions, except information that might identify individual beneficiaries, such as diagnosis codes and outlier payments, has been stripped. There is also a BEF for inpatient psychiatric stays, which is derived from the 2002 MedPAR data and cost report files. This is available on DVD and contains about 500,000 claims. It includes information about the facility used, such as type and size, as well as claims data.

Other Medicare Research Identifiable Files

Name and Address Files and *Vital Status Files* are subsets of the Enrollment Database and, on specific request, can be created by the CMS to support health care research. Two types of files can be created: one is based on a numeric search for records matching a list of social security numbers or Health Insurance Claim Numbers, and the other is based on drawing a demographic sample of enrollees. A Name and Address File contains beneficiary names and addresses, plus demographic information such as gender, race, date of birth, and date of death. CMS will create a Name and Address File only for the purpose of contacting beneficiaries for research and will not release the file to researchers. Instead, the researcher defines the sample, CMS creates the Name and Address File, and a CMS contractor mails information about the study to the individuals in the sample. A Vital Status File contains the same demographic information as a Name and Address File, but without beneficiary names and addresses; it is released directly to the researcher.

The *Renal Management Information System* (REMIS) stores information about ESRD patients. It replaced the previous system, REBUS, in July 2003. ESRD refers to complete or near-complete failure of kidney function, requiring dialysis or kidney transplantation; patients with ESRD have been included in the Medicare system since 1973. REMIS also determines Medicare coverage periods for ESRD and has access to both patient and facility data. Permission to use REMIS data must be reviewed by ResDAC. Once approved, the request can be submitted to CMS. Some ESRD facility- and provider-level information is available for download from the REMIS website (http://www.cms.hhs.gov/ESRDGeneralInformation/02_Data.asp#TopOfPage), including the 2004 facility survey data, file layout, and instructions, and the 2006 provider file and instructions.

The *Long Term Care Minimum Data Set* (LTCMDS or, for short, MDS) contains information about the physical, psychological, and psychosocial functioning of Medicare beneficiaries living in long-term care facilities. The MDS contains a subset of data from the screening and assessment elements of the Resident Assessment Instrument (RAI), which is used to assess a beneficiary's functioning when first admitted to a facility and periodically afterward. The RAI is normally administered quarterly, annually, when a serious error is discovered in a previous assessment, or when a beneficiary experiences a significant change in status. Because of the sensitive nature of these data, requests for MDS data must be made through the ResDAC. Further information about the MDS, including a *User's Manual* and the RAI form, is available for download at http://www.cms.hhs.gov/NursingHomeQualityInits/20_NHQIMDS20.asp.

Medicare Public Use Files

Medicare PUFs (also known as *Non-Identifiable Files*) do not contain information that would allow individuals to be identified. Most are summarized to levels higher than the individual. PUFs are in the public domain and are relatively inexpensive to order from CMS. Further information files are available from the CMS website at http://www. cms.hhs.gov/NonIdentifiableDataFiles/.

The *Health Care Information System* (HCIS) contains data from the SAFs summarized at various levels greater than the individual patient. The HCIS files include information from Medicare Part A (Inpatient, SNF, and Hospice), HHA (Part A and B), and Outpatient (Part B). Information available includes Medicare covered and noncovered days of care, Medicare payments, number of patients, and frequency of visits by type of service. HCIS data are available for each year from 2000 to 2004.

The *Part B Extract Summary System* (BESS) data file summarizes data about number of allowed services, amount of allowed charges, and payment amounts for Medicare Part B. BESS data are summarized from the Physician/Supplier Procedure Summary Master File. Two types of BESS files are available: the *BESS data file* is grouped by meaningful Healthcare Common Procedure Coding System/Current Procedural Terminology (HCPCS/CPT) code ranges, while the *BESS Carrier data file* is grouped by carrier and then by HCPCS/CPT code ranges. *Carrier* in this context means physician or other provider of services to Medicare beneficiaries. HCPCS/CPT code ranges group similar services or organ systems (e.g., Anesthesia, Respiratory, or Maternity). The BESS files include a total for each HCPCS/CPT code range, and break down into further categories and procedures. Further information is available from the BESS "Read Me" file available for download from http://www.cms.hhs. gov/NonIdentifiableDataFiles/Downloads/BESSCarrierReadme04.pdf. BESS data files are available on CD-ROM for the years 2000 to 2004; the BESS Carrier data file is available on CD-ROM for 2004.

The *Provider of Services* file (POS) contains information about nineteen types of Medicare-approved providers, including hospitals, SNFs, HHAs, rural health clinics, community mental health centers, and hospices. POS data are extracted from the Online Survey and Certification Reporting System database and include provider number, name, and address, plus characteristics of each provider such as the number and qualifications of personnel and number of beds. POS data are available on CD-ROM on a quarterly basis from 1991 through the current calendar quarter.

The *Hospital Service Area File* (HSAF) contains data about inpatient claims from institutions such as hospitals, rural health clinics, and community health centers, and is summarized by provider number and ZIP code of the Medicare beneficiary. Information contained in the HSAF includes total days of care, total charges, and total cases. HSAFs are available on CD-ROM for the years 1992 to 2005. Data are usually available in May for the previous year.

The *Physician/Supplier Procedure Summary Master File* is a summary of Part B Carrier and Durable Medical Equipment Regional Carrier claims. The summarized fields are total submitted services and charges, total allowed services and charges, total denied services and charges, and total payment amounts. These files are available for the years 1991 to 2004 and have been divided into twenty-four segments, by HCPCS range. The Physician/Supplier Procedure Summary Master File is produced annually and is generally available in July of the following year.

The *Unique Physician Identification Number* (UPIN) Directory contains information about physicians, doctors of osteopathy, and other types of practitioners enrolled in the Medicare program. Data are extracted from the UPIN database and includes the UPIN, full name, specialty, Physician License State Code, ZIP code, Medicare provider billing number, and state. The UPIN is currently the CMS provider identification number; however, it will no longer be used after the 4th Quarter 2006 Update and will be replaced by the National Provider Identifier (NPI). The UPIN Directory is available on CD-ROM and may also be searched online at the UPIN Registry website (http://www.upinregistry.com/).

The Medicare Current Beneficiary Survey

The MCBS has been conducted continuously since 1991, using a panel design to survey a nationally representative sample of Medicare beneficiaries for people who are elderly, who have disabilities, and who are institutionalized. It is the only comprehensive source of survey information concerning Medicare beneficiaries. Information collected by the MCBS includes demographic and socioeconomic characteristics, health status and functioning, health care utilization and expenditures, and health insurance coverage.

Focus

The goals of the MCBS are to gather longitudinal information on Medicare beneficiaries, including health services utilization, expenditures, insurance coverage, sources of payment, health status and functioning, and demographic and behavioral information. MCBS data are contained in two files that are released annually: the *Access to Care* file and the *Cost and Use* file. The Access to Care file contains information collected from individuals who were enrolled for the entire year (excluding those who entered the program during the year or who died during the year). The Cost and Use file includes most of the information from the Access to Care file plus reconciled cost and use information, and includes data for all people who were enrolled in Medicare for any part of the year.

Data Collection

The MCBS is conducted by Westat under contract with CMS. The MCBS sample is drawn from the CMS Medicare enrollment file in a two-stage process: geographic PSUs are selected, and a systematic random sample within age strata is selected within the PSUs. Geographic areas with large increases of persons age 65 and older since the 1980 U.S. Census are oversampled, as are persons with disabilities and those 85 years of age or older. The MCBS sample is sufficient to allow subgroup analyses by gender, region, and metropolitan/nonmetropolitan area, but not by race/ethnicity or smaller geographic regions such as state. Interview subjects are selected without regard to whether they live in a private residence or an institution, and interviews are conducted in the respondent's residence. Different questionnaire forms are used for community-dwelling individuals versus those living in long-term care facilities. If a selected individual is unable to answer the survey questions, a proxy respondent, usually a relative or close acquaintance, is used. About 15 percent of community interviews use proxy respondents, and all interviews for individuals living in long-term care facilities are conducted with proxy respondents.

MCBS interviews are conducted continuously, using a rotating panel design. Interviews are conducted in person using CAPI. Respondents are interviewed about every 4 months, and new respondents are added to the sample annually during the September–December round, to replenish cells depleted by deaths or refusals. MCBS began as a fixed-panel design with no limit on how long respondents would remain in the survey. However, the cumulative effect of nonresponse led to the decision in 1993 to limit future panels to 4 years, and the transition to a rotating panel design was complete by 1997. Currently, about one-third of the current sample is retired each fall, and approximately 6000 new respondents are added.

Data from respondents living in the community are gathered using the *Community Questionnaire*, which consists of core and supplemental questions. Core questions are asked at each interview, and cover the topics of household composition, health insurance, health care utilization since the last interview, and charges and payments for health care. Supplementary questions are asked only on an annual basis, and include demographic information, income and assets, access to care, satisfaction with care, health status and functioning, and usual source of care. Another type of supplemental question is included only episodically. A list of supplements included by round is available at http://www.cms.hhs.gov/apps/mcbs/COMsupl.asp.

Information about sampled individuals living in long-term care facilities is gathered using the *Facility Questionnaire*, which is similar to but shorter than the Community Questionnaire and is always conducted with proxy respondents. Typically, for a given beneficiary, questions about medical treatment and physical functioning would be answered by the individual's primary caregivers, and questions about charges and payments for care would be answered by facility administrative staff. The facility core questions include the beneficiary's history, use of heath care and medications, and charges and payments. The supplemental annual questions include demographics, health status, and insurance coverage. Selected information on facilities, including type, size, ownership, and level of facilities, is also collected annually. Response rates for initial community interviews are more than 80 percent, and for follow-up interviews more than 95 percent. Response rates for facility interviews are nearly 100 percent.

MCBS interview data are linked to Medicare claims and other administrative data, so the final file consists of survey, administrative, and claims data with personal identifying information removed. Conflicting information from the survey and claims files (i.e., if care events are reported in one but not the other) are reconciled using a series of rules. Further information is available from the CMS website at http://www.cms.hhs.gov/apps/mcbs/Linkage.asp.

Accessing Data and Ancillary Materials

The Access to Care file is intended to provide early access to MCBS data and is released within a year of each survey. It includes information about insurance coverage, health status and functioning, access to care, information needs, income, satisfaction with care, and summaries of use and expenditures, but does not include reconciled cost and use information. The Cost and Use file includes more detailed data, including reconciled cost and use information, and is released within 2 years of each survey. It links survey data with Medicare claims information and provides expenditure and source of payment information for all health care services (not merely those covered by Medicare). In addition, the Access to Care file represents the "always enrolled" Medicare population (i.e., those who were enrolled for the entire year), while the Cost and Use file represents the "ever enrolled" Medicare population (i.e., those who were enrolled for as little as 1 day during the year).

MCBS data are available for purchase from CMS for the years as EDCDIC files on tape. Access to Care files are available for the years 1991 to 2003, and Cost and Use files are available for the years 1992 to 2002. Further information is available from the CMS website (http://www.cms.hhs.gov/apps/mcbs/FileAval.asp). MCBS questionnaires are available for the years 1991 to 2004 on the CMS website at http://www.cms.hhs.gov/apps/mcbs/Quests.asp. All Community and Facility questionnaires for the years 1997 to 2004 are in CAPI format, while Facility data for the years 1991 to 1996 were collected using pencil-and-paper questionnaires.

The Medicare Health Outcomes Survey

The HOS began in 1998 as part of the HEDIS. It was the first outcomes measure used to determine the quality of care provided by Medicare managed care health plans, currently known as *Medicare Advantage* (MA) plans. The HOS was developed jointly by CMS and the National Committee for Quality Assurance and is administered by approved private survey vendors. The HOS collects data at baseline and 2-year follow-up on a sample of individuals covered by each MA plan, and remains the largest survey effort undertaken by CMS.

Focus

The HOS evaluates the success of Medicare managed care plans in maintaining or improving the physical and mental functioning over a 2-year period of Medicare beneficiaries. HOS data for each plan are used to compute Performance Measurement results, which are based on differences in functioning for plan beneficiaries between baseline and 2-year follow-up (categorized as better than, the same as, or worse than expected). Beneficiary functioning is evaluated using two scales, the Physical Component Summary (PCS) and Mental Component Summary (MCS), derived from the SF-36, a widely used survey that collects information about self-rated health and activity limitations. Performance measurement results are computed using a set of case mix/risk adjustment factors and adjusted for the fact that the mental and physical functioning of persons who are elderly is expected to decline over time.

Data Collection

Each MA plan is required to participate in the HOS. A random sample of individuals within each plan is selected at baseline and followed up after 2 years. Individuals are eligible to be selected for the HOS if they have been enrolled in the plan for at least 6 months and do not have ESRD. One thousand individuals per plan are selected if possible, and all plan beneficiaries are selected if MA enrollment is less than 1000.

The HOS is administered annually by mail survey, with telephone follow-ups using CATI if questionnaires are not returned or are incomplete. Questionnaires have changed over the years. The current survey consists of the SF-36 Health Survey and additional questions on demographics, health status and functioning, and morbidity. PCS and MCS scores derived from the SF-36 are used as the principal measure of a beneficiary's physical and mental functioning. Demographic and other information is collected partly to compute the risk adjustment for each plan. Information collected includes age, gender, race, education, marital status, and household income; chronic medical conditions; ability to perform activities of daily living; depression; and healthy days.

Accessing Data and Ancillary Materials

HOS data are released annually and are classified by cohort. For instance, Cohort I consists of the respondents for whom baseline data were collected in 1998 and for whom follow-up data were collected in 2000. HOS public-use files, which have been stripped of information to allow the identification of any particular beneficiary or plan, can be downloaded in ASCII format from the HOS website at http://www.hosonline. org/surveys/hos/hosdata.asp. HOS data are also available as BEFs and RIFs, which contain information that could identify a plan and/or an individual. The researcher must apply to CMS to use these files. Further information is available from the HOS website. Ancillary information available for HOS data includes *Data User's Guides* for each year and SAS code to translate the ASCII data to an SAS file. The HOS survey instruments for the years 1998 to 2006 are available for download from the HOS website at http://www.hosonline.org/surveys/hos/hosinstrument.asp.

Medicaid Data

Although they were created at the same time and are often confused because of the similarity in their names, there are fundamental differences between Medicaid and Medicare of which researchers should be cognizant. The most important difference between Medicaid and Medicare is that Medicaid eligibility and benefits are determined by each state, and both may change frequently, while Medicare is a federal entitlement program with straightforward and fairly consistent eligibility rules. In fact, most Medicare enrollees are eligible because of their age; in most cases, once an individual is eligible for Medicare, he or she remains eligible. This is in contrast to Medicaid, where an individual's status may change from eligible to ineligible several times in a single year, depending on income, employment situation, and state of residence. These facts mean that any use of Medicaid data to represent either the health care received by an individual in a given time period, or to make comparisons of utilization across states, is more complicated than such comparisons would be if Medicare data were used. In addition, most individuals eligible for Medicare are enrolled in the program, which is not always the case for Medicaid. For this reason, services used by Medicaid recipients should not automatically be assumed to represent services used or required by the poor.

The principal Medicaid data sets of interest to researchers are contained in the State Medicaid Research Files (SMRFs) for the years 1992 to 1998 and the Medicaid Analytic Extract (MAX) files for the year 1999 and on. Both the SMRFs and the MAX files contain Medicaid enrollment and utilization data, and both include information that would allow the identification of individual beneficiaries and physicians. They are both therefore classified as RIFs, and researchers must submit an application to the CMS for permission to use these data. SMRFs were created only for those states (approximately thirty) that elected to participate in electronic data submission or in the Medicaid Statistical Information System (MSIS), whereas MAX files are created for all fifty states and the District of Columbia.

File type and structure are similar for SMRFs and MAX files. There is one person-level file and four claims-level files; the claims-level files are based on *final action claims*, meaning claims for which all necessary adjustments have been made and errors resolved. The *Personal Summary File* is an "ever-enrolled" person-level file containing one record for each person enrolled in Medicaid for a least a single day in the year in question. It contains demographics (e.g., gender, race, date of birth), basis of eligibility, a summary of services used, monthly enrollment status, and maintenance assistance status. The *Inpatient File* contains claims records for enrollees who used inpatient services during the year. The SMRF includes two diagnostic fields and two procedure fields, while MAX files include ten diagnosis fields and seven procedure fields. Other information on the Inpatient File includes length of stay, payment amount, and discharge status. The *Long Term Care File* contains claims for long-term care services provided by SNFs, intermediate care facilities, and independent psychiatric facilities. The SMRF Long Term Care File includes one diagnostic field and no procedure fields, while MAX files include five diagnosis fields. Other data include facility type, discharge status, and dates of service. The *Drug File* contains drug claims and includes one procedure field. Since 1996, the Drug File has included the National Drug Code (NDC), whereas prior to that time both NDCs and HCPCS codes were used. The *Other Therapy File* contains claims for noninstitutional Medicaid services, including laboratory, x-ray, and physician and clinic services. Information available for a claim includes the diagnosis, procedure, and date of service. The SMRF included one diagnostic field and one procedure field, while MAX files include two diagnostic fields and one procedure field.

Individual beneficiaries are identified within SMRF and MAX files by their *Eligible Identification Number,* which appears in all five files and can be used to combine information about different types of services used by an individual.

Not all states participated in MSIS before 1999. A list of states and the years SMRF data are available for them is available from the ResDAC website at http://www.resdac.umn.edu/Medicaid/medicaidFAQ.asp. For the other states, Medicaid data files may be available directly from each state. MAX data for all states and the District of Columbia is currently available for 1999, 2000, and 2001. SMFR and MAX files are available only as tape cartridges.

Some Medicaid data are available in PUFs, which have been stripped of information that could identify individuals and are generally available only at levels of aggregation higher than the individual. State-level tabular data for the years 1999 to 2003 may be downloaded from http://www.cms.hhs.gov/medicaiddatasourcesgeninfo/02_msisdata.asp?.

National and state-specific data about drug utilization under the Medicaid Drug Rebate Program is available for download from http://www.cms.hhs.gov/MedicaidDrugRebateProgram/SDUD/list.asp. This file includes the NDC, number of prescriptions, number of units reimbursed, and total reimbursed amounts for each drug. Information about the Drug Rebate Program file, including the file layout and data definitions, is available for download from http://www.cms.hhs.gov/medicaiddrugrebateprogram/SDUD/list.asp.

Detailed information about Medicaid pharmacy benefit use in 1999 is available in a series of tables created by Mathematica Policy Research, Inc. (MPR), under contract from CMS. MPR used the MAX files and other data to create the *Statistical Compendium: Medicaid Pharmacy Benefit Use and Reimbursement in 1999*, a detailed series of tables at the national and state levels. An explanation of this project, and the tables themselves, are available at http://www.cms.hhs.gov/medicaiddatasourcesgeninfo/08_medicaidpharmacy.asp.

Other Sources of Data

This chapter discusses a number of data sources that may be of interest to the epidemiologist and public health researcher, although they are not focused exclusively on health issues. The U.S. Census is the basic source of demographic information about people living in the United States and is often used by health researchers to provide contextual information such as the racial makeup or economic status of geographic areas they are studying. The *Area Resource File* (ARF) contains health, economic, and demographic information drawn from a number of sources and aggregated at the county level. It is also frequently used to provide contextual information for geographic areas. The *General Social Survey* (GSS) is a telephone survey conducted since 1972 that collects data on a variety of social issues, including alcohol and drug use, sexual behavior, and attitudes toward health issues such as abortion and euthanasia. The ICPSR, located at the University of Michigan, is a repository of data on a variety of topics, many of which are health related, including data from the *Health and Medical Care Archive* (HMCA) of the Robert Wood Johnson Foundation (RWJF). The *Henry A. Murray Research Archive*, housed at Harvard University, contains data and ancillary materials from more than 270 longitudinal studies of human development and social change. The *Project on Human Development in Chicago Neighborhoods* (PHDCN) is a large-scale, longitudinal study of how child and adolescent development is affected by families, schools, and neighborhoods. *CDC WONDER*, *DataWeb*, and *FedStats* are web portals that allow access through the Internet to statistical information and data from a number of sources. Information about clinical trials is available through the *Adverse Event Reporting System*, the National Institutes of Health (NIH) website *ClinicalTrials.gov*, and the pharmaceutical industry clearinghouse website *ClincalStudyResults.org. StatLib,* the *Journal of the American Statistical Association Data Archive,* the *Data and Story Library* (DASL), and the *Time Series Data Library* are collections of data sets that are particularly useful for teaching statistics and data analysis.

The U.S. Census

The U.S. Census has been conducted every 10 years since 1790, in years ending with a "0" (e.g., 1790, 1800, 1810). Its primary purpose is to enumerate the population of the United States to allocate congressional seats, electoral votes, and government funding. However, the Census also collects information on topics such as income, education, and ethnicity, and is often used by public health researchers to provide contextual information for their research projects (i.e., to classify ZIP code areas by income level or housing cost). Because it is a census rather than a survey, it intends to collect information from every person living in the United States at the time of the Census, without regard to citizenship or immigration status. Although this might seem like a simple process, in reality there have been serious criticisms that certain people are excluded from the Census or are undercounted in a nonrandom fashion. In particular, some researchers argue that Census data do not fully represent two classes of people. The first potentially misrepresented class includes homeless or migratory individuals who may have been missed because the data collection plan for the Census is based on housing units. The second class includes poor, non-White people living in urban areas who have been undercounted for a variety of reasons, including nonstandard living arrangements and distrust of government officials. Some statisticians have argued that the Census Bureau could improve the accuracy by using modern sampling techniques and statistical adjustments to correct for such suspected undercounts, but to date this has not become official policy.

The questions included and data collection methods of the Census have varied over its history. The 2000 Census, which is the most recent available, relied on a combination of questionnaires mailed to individual residences, plus questionnaires personally delivered by Census enumerators for homes lacking street name and house number addresses (mostly in rural areas). The questionnaires were available in six languages: English, Spanish, Tagalog, Korean, Chinese, and Vietnamese. Special operations were conducted to count migratory laborers, the homeless, and those who lived in nonstandard housing such as institutions or group homes. Census workers also followed up by telephone or in person with households that did not respond to the mailed questionnaire.

Two forms were used to collect data for the 2000 Census. The short form, which was administered to every household, collected information on whether the housing unit was owned, rented, or vacant, plus the age, gender, race/ethnicity, and household relationship of each person living in the household. The long form, which was administered to a random sample of approximately one in six households, collected detailed information on a number of topics, including education, employment, income, ancestry, migration, languages spoken, and home value or rental costs. Concerns have been raised about the actual "randomness" of the sample used for the long form and whether data collected from that sample adequately represents the U.S. population.

Census data are collected from individual households and aggregated into a variety of nested units of differing sizes. Nesting means that all the lower-level units are contained within upper-level units so a set of census blocks are included in a specific block group, that block group is included with other block groups in a specific census tract, and so on. A detailed diagram of the Census geographic hierarchy, showing the nesting structure and different levels of aggregation, and definitions of each level of the hierarchy, is available from http://www.census.gov/geo/www/tiger/glossry2.pdf. The basic plan, with the largest division at the top and each subsequent level nested within the levels above, is

United States
Region
Division
State
County
County subdivision
Place (or part)
Census tract (or part)
Block group (or part)
Census block

Although Census data are collected at the individual level, because of confidentiality concerns, most Census files are available only at higher levels of aggregation. The primary exception is the Public Use Microdata Series (PUMS) files described here, which represent a sample from the main Census files. Data and documentation for the 1990 and 2000 Censuses are available for download from the "American FactFinder" section of the U.S. Census website (http://factfinder.census.gov/home/saff/main.html?_lang=en). In addition, this website includes an interactive interface that allows users to find information such as population or racial makeup for a specific state, county, city, or ZIP code. Data for previous Census years are available from the ICPSR website (http://www.icpsr.umich.edu).

Census 2000 information is contained in four Summary Files (SFs), referred to as SF1 through SF4. SF1 contains 286 tables focusing on age, gender, households, families, and housing units. Tables are broken down by race, Hispanic origin, American Indian and Alaska Native tribe, Asian ethnic group, and Native Hawaiian and Pacific Islander group. Data are included for the United States, the fifty states, and the District of Columbia in the hierarchical sequence noted previously; some tables are available down to the block level, and some only to the census tract level. Summaries by other geographic areas, such as ZIP code tabulation areas are also included. SF2 contains forty-seven tables focusing on age, gender, households, families, and occupied housing units, which are available for the total population and for 249 population groups. SF3 contains 813 tables of social, economic, and housing characteristics compiled from Census 2000 long-form data, based on a one-sixth sample of U.S. households. Tables are repeated for nine major racial and ethnic groups, and data are presented in the same hierarchical format used for SF1. SF4 contains data compiled from the questions asked of a sample of all people and housing units. Tables are repeated for 336 population groups, including racial, ethnic, and ancestry groups. Documentation for each file is available from http://www.census.gov/main/www/cen2000.html.

The American Community Survey (ACS) is an ongoing statistical survey that will replace the long form of the 2010 Census. The ACS began in 1996 and has been expanded each year since then. Ultimately, it will include the residents of more than 3 million housing units in every county in the United States. The ACS questionnaire and information about sampling and data collection procedures are available from the ACS website at http://www.census.gov/acs/www/SBasics/index.htm.

Census data are available at the individual level through the Integrated Public Use Microdata Series (IPUMS) data files, also called PUMS files, which consist of data sampled from the each surviving Census since 1850 (the 1890 Census data were destroyed in a fire) and the ACS for the years 2000 to 2004. Most samples are at the 1 percent level, although 5 percent samples are also available for 1980 to 2000. The IPUMS files contain most of the data collected by the Census or ACS, with the exception of name and address; other data that could identify an individual (e.g., very high income) are suppressed or truncated, and geographic identifiers are not released for areas with less than 100,000 inhabitants. IPUMS data, and further information about the IPUMS project, are available through the University of Minnesota IPUMS website (http://www.ipums.org/usa/index.html).

PUMS data and documentation for a 1 and 5 percent sample of Census 2000 data are also available from the U.S. Census website: http://www.census.gov/Press-Release/www/2003/PUMS.html (1 percent sample) and http://www.census.gov/Press-Release/www/2003/PUMS5.html (5 percent sample). Data are available for each state, the District of Columbia, and Puerto Rico.

The Area Resource File

The ARF is a database containing information drawn from a number of sources, including data collected by the U.S. Census Bureau, the Bureau of Labor Statistics, the American Medical Association, the American Hospital Association, the NCHS, and the CMS. The ARF collects into a single database a variety of information useful for researchers, planners, and policy makers interested in health care delivery and factors that influence health status and health care in the United States. Although much of the information contained in the ARF is available elsewhere, it is often used by health researchers for reasons of convenience. The ARF is organized at the county level and contains a number of standard geographic identifiers that facilitate analysis at different levels of aggregation and allow ARF information to be merged with data from other files containing geographic identifiers.

The ARF includes data in three general categories: health care professions; hospitals and health care facilities; and demographic, environmental, and geographic information. *Health care professions* information includes detailed information on physicians, including age, gender, specialty, major professional activity, and graduation location; information about the number of other health care professionals, including dentists, veterinarians, optometrists, nurses, psychologists, and social workers; health professions shortage areas; and enrollment and graduation numbers for schools that educate health professionals, including medical schools, dental schools, pharmacy schools, and nursing schools. *Hospital and health care facilities* data include size, personnel, and number of admissions, inpatient days, outpatient visits, discharges, and ED visits for hospitals and nursing care facilities; numbers of different types of institutions, including rural health clinics, ambulatory surgery centers, home health agencies, community mental health centers; Health Maintenance Organization enrollment; hospital expenditures; and Medicare enrollment and reimbursement. *Demographic, environmental, and geographic* data include age, race, and gender in Census years and total population for intervening years; mortality, infant mortality, and natality; civilian employment and unemployment; income; housing density; land area; state and county codes; and metropolitan statistical area designations.

Each year a new ARF is released that includes the data for the immediately preceding year plus all previous years (as far back as 1970 for some variables); for instance, the 2005 file includes data through 2004. Not all data are available for every year included in the ARF. Information about what information is available for which years may be obtained through a search engine available from the ARF website (http://www.arfsys.com/). ARF data may be purchased from Quality Resource Systems, Inc., and more information on this can be found on the ARF website. The 2005 ARF data are available in two forms: as an ASCII file on CD-ROM or as a Microsoft Access database that includes an interface allowing the user to extract data to Access or Excel files. It is also possible to purchase a custom subset of ARF data from Quality Resource Systems; such data can be provided in several formats.

The General Social Survey

The GSS is a telephone survey that collects information from a probability sample of American households on a broad range of topics of interest to social science researchers. The first GSS was conducted in 1972, and it was conducted annually, with the exception of the years 1979, 1981, and 1992, until 1994; since 1994, it has been conducted every other year. Although different households are surveyed each year, the GSS questionnaires are designed to allow the study of change over time through the replication of individual items and item sequences. The GSS is conducted by the National Opinion Research Center, a research center affiliated with the University of Chicago.

GSS questions cover a variety of subjects, including demographics, behaviors, and attitudes. Researchers looking for data on a particular topic may use the subject index and search facility available on the ICPSR website (http://www.icpsr.umich.edu). General subject queries are matched with specific questions dealing with that topic, and each question is linked to a chart showing the years it was included in the survey, and responses by year and cumulatively. Many GSS topics may be of interest to public health researchers, including health, mental health, sexuality and sexual behaviors, social networks, attitudes toward medical care, and use of and attitudes toward tobacco, alcohol, and drugs.

The GSS is administered to about 3000 subjects annually, with a response rate of 70 to 75 percent. A cumulative file of GSS data for the years 1972 to 2004 may be downloaded from the University of California at Berkeley website (http://sda.berkeley.edu/archive.htm), and the cumulative codebook may be downloaded from the ICPSR website. The cumulative data file on CD-ROM and a hard copy of the codebook may also be purchased from the Roper Center at the University of Connecticut (http://www.ropercenter.uconn.edu/gss.html). GSS data and ancillary information for individual years are also available from the ICPSR website. General information about the GSS and a bibliography of publications using GSS data are available from the GSS website (http://www.norc.uchicago.edu/projects/gensoc.asp). Detailed information about sampling procedures is available from the ICPSR website at http://webapp.icpsr.umich.edu/GSS/rnd1998/appendix/apdx_a.htm.

The Inter-university Consortium for Political and Social Research

The ICPSR, located at the University of Michigan, maintains and provides access to an archive of social science data that includes many data sets of interest to public health researchers. ICPSR is a membership organization (more than 500 universities and colleges are currently members), so although some ICPSR data are freely available to members of the general public, other data sets are available only to individuals at member institutions. Some ICPSR data are available only through download from the ICPSR website (http://www.icpsr.umich.edu), while other data are available in other formats such as CD-ROM. In addition, some ICPSR data are available elsewhere (e.g., Census data), and some is unique to ICPSR. All ICPSR documentation is available for free download through the ICPSR website (http://www.icpsr.umich.edu/). This documentation is often substantial, including codebooks, computer syntax, user's guides, and bibliographies of articles that used a particular data set.

The ICPSR website offers several ways to locate data sets of interest, including a search mechanism and topical lists. A search on the topic "Health Care and Facilities" returned 493 data sets, which range from recent national polls on topics such as reproductive rights and genetic engineering to a file on the height and weight of West Point cadets for the second half of the nineteenth century. Data from many national surveys, such as the NHIS, NHANES, and U.S. Census are available from the ICPSR website. Even if a user prefers to access the data from the survey's web page, the documentation and related materials from the ICPSR website may be useful.

The HMCA is available through the ICPSR. It is the repository of data from research projects sponsored by the RWJF and includes more than sixty-five data collections. Primary topics include Cost and Access to Health Care, Substance Abuse and Health, Chronic Health Conditions, and Health Care Providers. The *Community Tracking Study* (CTS), a large-scale longitudinal investigation of health system change and its effects on people sponsored by the RWJF, may be of particular interest to public health researchers. The CTS began in 1996 and collects information in 2-year cycles, primarily through nationally representative surveys of households, physicians, and employers. The household survey gathers information about health status, limitations, health insurance, health care utilization, and quality of care. The physician survey gathers information about practice arrangements, sources of revenue, level of compensation, effects of care management strategies, allocation of time, provision of charity care, and career satisfaction. The employer survey gathers information about health insurance offered, employee eligibility and enrollment, and costs and benefits of each plan offered.

Most HMCA data may be downloaded only to researchers affiliated with ICPSR member institutions, but data from the CTS are available to anyone from the HMCA website, which is located within the ICPSR website (http://www.icpsr.umich.edu/HMCA/cts.html). In addition, two CD-ROMs containing data from the HMCA can be purchased through the ICPSR: one contains twenty-one data sets concerning a variety of health care topics, and the other contains data from the CTS and related studies. Further information about these CD-ROMs is available from http://www.icpsr.umich.edu/HMCA/cdrom.html.

Limited online analysis of some ICPSR data are possible through the Data Analysis System (DAS), which can be accessed through the ICPSR website at http://www.icpsr.umich.edu/access/sda.html. Currently, about 200 data sets are available for DAS, which allows the user to search for variables within a data set, create frequency tables and summary statistics, create statistical tables and graphs, recode variables and compute new variables, and create subsets of cases or variables for download. Most DAS components are available to all users; some are limited to users from ICPSR member institutions.

The Henry A. Murray Research Archive

The Henry A. Murray Research Archive, located at Harvard University, is a research archive concerned primarily with longitudinal studies of human development and social change, focusing particularly on issues of concern to women. The primary purpose of the Murray Archive is to make longitudinal data sets and other research materials, such as interview transcripts, videotapes, and audiotapes, available to researchers for secondary analysis. Ancillary materials relating to the data sets are also available from the archive, including questionnaires or other research instruments, descriptions of the data collection processing and coding procedures, and publications based on data stored in the archive.

The Murray Archive currently holds data from more than 270 studies and continues to accept new data sets. The holdings of the archive would be of particular interest to public health researchers interested in topics with a social or psychological aspect, such as the influence of social context on behavior, or the patterns of intellectual and personality development over time. Detailed information about many of the data sets available through the Murray Archive may be found in *Inventory of Longitudinal Studies in the Social Sciences* (Young, Savola, & Phelps, 1991), and there is also a search function and classified index available on the archive's website at http://vdc.hmdc.harvard.edu/VDC/. Searches are possible by topic and also by study sample characteristics, including sample size, age, gender, socioeconomic status, and race.

Researchers must apply for permission to use data from the Murray Archive. A form for this purpose is available from the archive website at http://murray.harvard.edu/mra/service.jsp?id=51&bct=dData percent2BAccess.s51. Once permission is granted, most materials may be used offsite, and some may be downloaded from the website.

The Project on Human Development in Chicago Neighborhoods

The PHDCN is a large-scale, interdisciplinary study of how child and adolescent development is affected by families, schools, and neighborhoods. Although public health was not the exclusive focus of the PHDCN, it collected data on many topics of interest to public health researchers, including adolescent substance abuse and antisocial behavior, and the influence of prenatal and postnatal conditions on infant growth and health. The PHDCN was directed by researchers from the Harvard School of Public Health and was conducted in Chicago because of the diversity of race, ethnicity, and social class in that city, and because of the stable nature of Chicago neighborhoods.

The PHDCN created 347 Neighborhood Clusters (NCs) with about 8000 residents each, by grouping together Census tracts. Definition of the NCs was partially informed by the history and culture of the areas (i.e., they attempted to accommodate residents' definitions of what constituted a neighborhood). NCs were also designed to be homogenous in socioeconomic status and racial/ethnic makeup, if those features typified the local definition of a given neighborhood. PHDCN data were collected over 8 years and include four separate components. Data for the *Community Survey* were collected twice, in 1994 to 1995 and 2001 to 2002, through household interviews conducted with randomly selected adults from all the NCs. Community Survey questions focused on social cohesion, social control, cultural values, and the organization and structure of each local community. The *Systematic Social Observation* component gathered information from eighty of the NCs through direct observation of neighborhoods one block at a time. Observations were coded to assess characteristics such as social interaction, graffiti, land use, housing, and litter. The *Longitudinal Cohort Study* selected random cohorts of children, adolescents, and young adults and their primary caregivers, and followed them over 7 years to track changes in their circumstances and personal characteristics. Data were collected in three waves, of which only Wave 1 (1994–1997) has currently been released. The *Infant Assessment Unit* studied in greater detail 412 infants and their primary caregivers included in Wave 1 of the *Longitudinal Cohort Study*. They were given an additional assessment at the age of 5 to 7 months, and were videotaped to capture infant–caregiver interaction and infant response to stimulation.

The release of PHDCN data through the ICPSR website (http://www.icpsr.umich.edu/PHDCN) is an ongoing process, owing to the large number and size of the data files involved. Almost 800 files are expected to be released by the end of 2006. Data are available in SAS, SPSS, and Stata formats, and documentation is in PDF format. Ancillary information available from the ICPSR website includes a description of the project, codebooks, detailed information about technical issues such as sampling methods and response rates, and bibliographies of publications using PHDCN data. Further information on the PHDCN is also available from the Harvard website for this project (http://www.hms.harvard.edu/chase/projects/chicago/).

Web Portals to Statistical Data

Three websites serve as portals through which a variety of health-related information and data can be retrieved. The *CDC WONDER* (Wide-ranging OnLine Data for Epidemiological Research) site (http://wonder.cdc.gov) provides convenient access to information from the CDC. The main advantage of using the CDC WONDER portal is that it allows the user to search a number of data sources and document collections simultaneously, or alternately to access information through alphabetical and topical indexes. CDC WONDER includes an online query system that allows the user to perform simple calculations and produce maps or reports on health-related topics (e.g., leading causes of death in Missouri for the years 1999 to 2002) without downloading data.

The *DataWeb* is a joint collaboration between the CDC and the U.S. Census Bureau that provides simultaneous access to a number of major data sets (currently, to fifteen) through a single portal. Data sets accessible through DataWeb include Census data for 1990 and 2000, the American Community Survey, the BRFSS, the NHIS, the Consumer Expenditure Survey, and the Survey of Income and Program Participation. A complete list of data sets included is available at http://www.thedataweb.org/datasets.html. The DataWeb may be accessed using *DataFerrett* (Federated Electronic Research, Review, Extraction and Tabulation Tool), free software available in Macintosh and Windows versions (including an Applet version), which may be downloaded from http://dataferrett.census.gov/index.html. Operations available through DataFerrett include computing statistics, producing tables and maps, and extracting and downloading data for further analysis.

FedStats (http://www.fedstats.gov/) provides an online interface with links to statistical information from more than 100 federal agencies. This website includes a topical index and search function. The primary usefulness of this website for epidemiologists and public health researchers is its ability to find health-related information from agencies that do not focus primarily on health. For instance, a search on "HIV" returned a link to 2002 and 2003 Bureau of Justice reports on HIV/AIDS in prisons.

Adverse Events and Clinical Trials Information

The U.S. Food and Drug Administration maintains the *Adverse Event Reporting System* (AERS), an information database containing information about adverse events reported for approved drug and therapeutic biological products. Drug manufacturers are required to report adverse events, and health care professionals and consumers have the option to do so. AERS data files in ASCII or SGML formats for the years 2004 to 2006 may be downloaded from the AERS website (http://www.fda.gov/cder/aers/default.htm). Older files may be purchased from the NTIS. Information is available at http://www.ntis.gov.

Consumer information about clinical trials (including both those conducted by governmental agencies and by the pharmaceutical industry) accessed through the NIH website *ClincalTrials.gov* (http://www.clinicaltrials.gov/). This website includes information about the clinical trials process, listings of clinical trials by condition, sponsor, and status, and a search engine. The primary purpose of ClincalTrials.gov is to allow people to locate clinical trials for which they may be eligible. Information provided for each trial includes a detailed description of the trial, location, eligibility, study status (i.e., if they are currently recruiting), the ClinicalTrials.gov identifier number, and contact information. Data sets are not available through this interface.

The Pharmaceutical Research and Manufacturers of America database available through the *ClincalStudyResults.org* website provides information about clinical trials. Both company-provided information and references or links to published articles are included. The primary audience is physicians, and the information provided is more technical than that available through ClinicalTrials.gov. A search engine is available at http://www.clinicalstudyresults.org/home/ that provides access by company name, condition or disease, generic name, brand name, and indication. Participation in the ClincalStudyResults.org database is voluntary, so it should not be considered an exhaustive resource. Data are not available through this database.

Data Sets Commonly Used in Teaching

The data sets discussed in this section are available for download from the Internet and are often used in teaching statistics classes. In some cases, these data sets have been made available by the individuals whose research they represent, and they are often accompanied by information about the research project from which they are drawn, such as the data collection and analysis process, and include references or links to published articles using the data.

Carnegie Mellon University maintains three websites that provide access to a number of data sets that can be freely downloaded and analyzed. The main website is called *StatLib* (http://lib.stat.cmu.edu/index.php) and includes more than 100 data sets. Some of the data sets included at this website are electronic versions of the data used in popular statistical textbooks, and others are data from research projects that illustrate interesting points, often accompanied by suggestions of how they can be used to illustrate particular topics or techniques in statistics classes. Many topic areas are represented in the data sets. Those relevant to public health include comparisons of the estimation of body fat by various methods, the relationship between arsenic in well water and as deposited in people's bodies, and deaths within 30 days of heart transplant surgery at different hospitals.

Carnegie Mellon is also the principal site for access to the data archive for articles published in the *Journal of the American Statistical Association*. This archive may be accessed from http://lib.stat.cmu.edu/jasadata/. This is a smaller archive and is focused more on data that will support advanced statistical techniques. The supporting information is similar to that in the main StatLib archive, and several of the data sets concern public health topics, including nutrient intake, HIV transmission, and smoking trends.

The DASL is the third major data resource available from StatLib. The DASL website is http://lib.stat.cmu.edu/DASL/. As the name suggests, DASL consists of stories (i.e., prose narratives centered on particular topics), plus data files related to the stories and suggestions for exploration and analysis of the data. The stories and data sets are searchable by name, method (e.g., correlation, linear regression), and topic (e.g., health, medicine). Each data set includes a statement as to whether it is completely in the public domain, or whether it may be used for teaching purposes but not for publication.

The *Time Series Data Library* was created by Rob Hyndman and is maintained at Monash University. It contains more than 800 time series data sets in text format, which can be downloaded from http://www.personal.buseco.monash.edu.au/~hyndman/TSDL/. All data files are referenced to a source, most often a published article or textbook. Although the data sets included in the *Time Series Data Library* are often available elsewhere, it is a convenient collection of time series data sets in electronic format from a variety of fields of study. Examples of public health topics covered by the data sets include monthly cases of chickenpox in New York City for the years 1931 to 1972, annual fertility rates in Sweden for the years 1750 to 1849, and annual suicide rates in the United States for the years 1920 to 1969.

Acronyms

Acronym	Full name (relevant data set, program, or agency)
ACIP	Advisory Committee on Immunization Practices (NIS)
ACS	American Community Survey (Census Bureau)
AERS	Adverse Event Reporting System (FDA)
AHRQ	Agency for Healthcare Research and Quality (MEPS, HCUP)
APC	Ambulatory Payment Classification (CMS)
ARF	Area Resource File
ASCII	American Standard Code for Information Interchange
BEF	Beneficiary Encrypted File (Medicare)
BESS	Part B Extract Summary System (Medicare)
BRFSS	Behavior Risk Factor Surveillance System
CAPI	Computer-Assisted Personal Interviewing
CATI	Computer-Assisted Telephone Interviewing
CDC	Centers for Disease Control and Prevention
CII	Childhood Immunization Initiative (NIS 1)
CMF	Compressed Mortality File
CMS (1)	Centers for Medicare and Medicaid Services
CMS (2)	Current Mortality Sample
CTS	Community Tracking Study (HMCA)
DRG	Diagnosis-Related Group (Medicare)
ED	Emergency Department
ESRD	End-Stage Renal Disease

(Continued)

Acronym	Full name (relevant data set, program, or agency)
FIPS	Federal Information Processing Standards (ARF, U.S. Census)
FSASC	Free-standing ambulatory surgery center (NSAS)
FTP	File Transfer Protocol
GPO	Government Printing Office
GSS	General Social Survey
HC	Household Component (MEPS)
HCIS	Health Care Information System (Medicare)
HCPCS/CPT	Healthcare Common Procedure Coding System/ Current Procedural Terminology (Medicaid)
HCUP	Healthcare Cost and Utilization Project
HHANES	Hispanic Health and Nutrition Examination Survey
HMCA	Health and Medical Care Archive (ICPSR)
HOS	Health Outcomes Survey (Medicare)
HSAF	Hospital Service Area File (Medicare)
IC	Insurance Component (MEPS)
ICD	International Classification of Diseases
ICPSR	Inter-university Consortium for Political and Social Research
IPUMS	Integrated Public Use Microdata Series (U.S. Census)
JCUSH	Joint Canada/United States Survey of Health
KID	Kids' Inpatient Database (HCUP)
LDS	Limited Data Set (Medicare)
LF	Longitudinal Followup (NMIHS)
LSOA	Longitudinal Studies of Aging
LTCH	Long Term Care Hospital
LTMCMDS	Long Term Care Minimum Data Set (same as MDS) (Medicare)
MA	Medicare Advantage
MAX	Medicaid Analytic Extract
MCBS	Medicare Current Beneficiary Summary
MDS	Minimum Data Set (same as LTCMDS) (Medicare)
MedPAR	Medicare Provider Analysis and Review

Acronym	Full name (relevant data set, program, or agency)
MEPS	Medical Expenditures Panel Survey
MMWR	*Morbidity and Mortality Weekly Report*
MPC	Medical Provider Component (MEPS)
MSIS	Medicaid Statistical Information System
MTF	Monitoring the Future
NAACCR	North American Association of Central Cancer Registries (SEER)
NAMCS	National Ambulatory Medical Care Survey
NC	Neighborhood Cluster (PHDCN)
NCHS	National Center for Health Statistics
NCI	National Cancer Institute
NCQA	National Committee for Quality Assurance (Medicare)
NDC	National Drug Code
NDI	National Death Index
NEHIS	National Employer Health Insurance Survey (MEPS)
NHAMCS	National Hospital Ambulatory Medical Care Survey
NHANES	National Health and Nutrition Examination Survey
NHC	Nursing Home Component (MEPS)
NHDS	National Hospital Discharge Survey
NHES	National Health Examination Survey
NHHCS	National Home and Hospice Care Survey
NHIS	National Health Interview Survey
NHPI	National Health Provider Inventory
NIA	National Institute on Aging
NIH	National Institutes of Health
NIS (1)	National Immunization Survey
NIS (2)	Nationwide Inpatient Sample (HCUP)
NMFS	National Mortality Followback Study
NMIHS	National Maternal and Infant Health Survey
NNHS	National Nursing Home Survey
NNSS	National Nutritional Surveillance System
NPI	National Provider Inventory (Medicare)
NSAS	National Survey of Ambulatory Surgery

(*Continued*)

Acronym	Full name (relevant data set, program, or agency)
NSFG	National Survey of Family Growth
NTIS	National Technical Information Service
NVSS	National Vital Statistics System
OPD	Outpatient Department
OPPS	Outpatient Prospective Payment System (Medicare)
PHDCN	Project on Human Development in Chicago Neighborhoods
PHP	Partial Hospitalization Program (Medicare)
POS	Provider of Services (Medicare)
PPS	Prospective Payment System (Medicare)
PRAMS	Pregnancy Risk Assessment Monitoring System
PRC	Provider Record Check (NIS 1)
PSU	Primary Sampling Unit
PUF	Public Use File (Medicare)
RDC	Research Data Center (NCHS)
REMIS	Renal Management Information System (Medicare)
ResDAC	Research Data Assistance Center (CMS)
RIF	Research Identifiable File (Medicare)
SAF	Standard Analytical File (Medicare)
SASD	State Ambulatory Surgery Databases (HCUP)
SEDD	State Emergency Department Database (HCUP)
SEER	Surveillance Epidemiology and End Results
SID	State Inpatient Databases (HCUP)
SLAITS	State and Local Area Integrated Telephone Survey
SMRF	State Medicaid Research Files
SNF	Skilled Nursing Facility
SOA	Supplement on Aging (LSOA)
UPIN	Unique Physician Identification Number (Medicare)
YRBSS	Youth Risk Behavior Survey Surveillance System

Summary of Data Sets
and Years Available

Title	Focus	Years (data available)
Chapter 2		
National Health Care Survey		
National Ambulatory Medical Care Survey	Physician office visits	1973–1981, 1985, 1989–(annual)
National Hospital Ambulatory Medical Care Survey	Hospital outpatient department and emergency department visits	1992–(annual)
National Hospital Discharge Survey	Inpatient hospital stays	1965–(annual)
National Nursing Home Survey	Nursing home facilities and residents	1973–1974, 1977, 1985, 1995, 1999, 2003
National Health Provider Inventory	Health care providers	1991
National Survey of Ambulatory Surgery	Ambulatory surgery visits	1994, 1995, 1996
National Home and Hospice Care Survey	Home health care agencies and hospices and their residents	1992, 1993, 1994, 1996, 1998, 2000
National Employer Health Insurance Survey	Employer-sponsored health insurance	1994
The Healthcare Cost and Utilization Project		(availability may vary by state)
The State Inpatient Databases	Inpatient hospital stays	1990–2004
The State Ambulatory Surgery Databases	Ambulatory surgery visits	1997–2004
The State Emergency Department Databases	ED visits	1997–2004
The Nationwide Inpatient Sample	Inpatient hospital stays	1988–2003
The Kids' Inpatient Database	Child inpatient hospital stays	1988–2003
Medical Expenditures Panel Survey	Health care utilization and costs	1996–(annual)
National Immunization Survey	Child (19–35 months) immunization	1992–(annual)

(Continued)

(*Continued*)

Title	Focus	Years (data available)
Surveillance Epidemiology and End Results	Cancer	1973–(annual)
Chapter 3		
Behavior Risk Factor Surveillance System	Adult health risk behaviors	1984–(annual)
Youth Risk Behavior Surveillance System	Youth (9th–12th grades) health risk behaviors	1992–(even-numbered years)
Monitoring the Future	Youth (8th, 10th, and 12th grades) drug, alcohol, and tobacco use	1975–(annual)
Chapter 4		
National Health Examination Survey	Health	1960–1962, 1963–1965, 1966–1970
National Health and Nutrition Examination Survey	Health and nutrition	1971–1975, 1976–1980, 1982–1984, 1988–1994, 1999–(annual)
Hispanic Health and Nutrition Examination Survey	Health among Hispanic Americans	1982–1984
National Health Interview Survey	Health	1957–(annual)
Joint Canada/United States Survey of Health	Health and health care access	2002–2003
Longitudinal Studies of Aging	Health of older adults (age 70+)	1984–1990, 1994–2000 (every other year)
State and Local Area Integrated Telephone Survey		
Health Module	Health	1997
Child Well-Being and Welfare Module	Child well-being and participation in public assistance programs	1998–1999
National Survey of Early Childhood Health	Child (age 4–35 months) health	2000
National Survey of Children with Special Health Care Needs	Prevalence and impact of children with special health care needs	2001, 2005–2006
National Survey of Children's Health	Health of children (age 0–17 years)	2003–2004
National Asthma Survey	Asthma control and care	2003–2004
Chapter 5		
The National Vital Statistics System		
Public-Use Natality Files	Births	1968–(annual)
Public-Use Mortality Files	Deaths	1968–(annual)

Title	Focus	Years (data available)
Public-Use Fetal Death Files	Fetal deaths	1982–1995
Perinatal Mortality Data Set	Births, infant deaths, and fetal deaths	1995–1999
Linked Birth and Infant Death Files	Children who died at <1 year of age	1983–1991, 1995–2002
Public-Use Marriage Files	Marriages	1968–1990
Public-Use Divorce Files	Divorces	1968–1990
Compressed Mortality File	Deaths (aggregated to county level)	1968–2002
National Death Index	Death records	1979–2004
National Mortality Followback Study	Various (supplements death certificate information)	1962–1963, 1964–1965, 1966–1968, 1986, 1993
National Maternal and Infant Health Survey and Longitudinal Followup	Adverse pregnancy outcomes	1988 (NMIHS), 1991 (LF)
Pregnancy Risk Assessment Monitoring System	Adverse birth outcomes	1987–(annual)
National Survey of Family Growth	Fertility, marriage, sexual behavior, maternal and infant health	1973, 1976, 1982, 1988, 1995, 2002
Chapter 6		
Medicare Administrative Files		
Denominator Record Files	Demographic and enrollment information	1991–2005
Standard Analytical Files	Medicare Part A and Part B claims	1991–2004
Medicare Provider Analysis and Review Files	Inpatient hospital and skilled nursing facility claims	1991–2003
Prospective Payment System Files	Outpatient and Partial Hospitalization Program claims	2004
Renal Management Information System	End-stage renal disease patients	2003–(annual)
Long Term Care Minimum Data Set	Functioning of residents of long-term care facilities	N/A
Health Care Information System	Summarized Medicare Part A and Part B claims	2000–2004
Part B Extract Summary System	Summarized Part B claims	2000–2004
Provider of Services File	Health care institutions (hospitals, skilled nursing facilities, home health agencies, etc.)	1991–(quarterly)

(Continued)

(*Continued*)

Title	Focus	Years (data available)
Hospital Service Area File	Summarized inpatient claims	1992–2005
Physician/Supplier Procedure Summary Master File	Summarized claims for physician services and medical equipment	1991–2004
Unique Physician Identification Number Directory	Physicians	Current (updated quarterly)
Medicare Current Beneficiary Survey	Health status and health care	1991–(annual)
Medicare Health Outcomes Survey	Physical and mental functioning of enrollees of Medicaid managed care plans	1998–(annual)
Medicaid Data		
State Medicaid Research Files	Medicaid enrollment and claims	1992–1998
Medicaid Analytic Extract	Medicaid enrollment and claims	1999–(annual)
Chapter 7		
U.S. Census	Demographics, housing	1850–2004
Area Resource File	Demographics, health care	1970–(updated annually)
General Social Survey	Social attitudes and behaviors	1972–1978, 1980, 1980–1991, 1993, 1994–(every other year)
Inter-university Consortium for Political and Social Research	Varied (data archive)	Varies
Henry A. Murray Research Archive	Longitudinal data	Varies
Project on Human Development in Chicago Neighborhoods	Child development, environment	Varies
Adverse Events Reporting System	Adverse reactions to drugs	2004–2006
StatLib	Teaching introductory statistics	Varies
JASA Data Archive	Teaching advanced statistics	Varies
Data and Story Library	Teaching introductory statistics	Varies
Time Series Data Library	Teaching time series methods	Varies

Data Import and Transfer

Many of the data sets discussed in this volume are provided in ASCII (plain text) format or another nonspecific format such as comma-separated or tab-delimited values. However, analysis of these data will usually be performed using a proprietary statistical analysis package such as SAS, SPSS, or Stata, which requires that the data be imported into that program and translated to the format it favors. There are several ways to get data from the supplied format to that required by a particular statistical package. One is to use the import facility or "wizard" that many statistical packages now include; this allows the user to import and translate data through an interactive interface. Another way is to use a program written to translate data from one format to another, such as Stat/Transfer, which can read and write data in about thirty different formats. Further information on Stat/Transfer, including a download-able trial copy, is available from www.stattransfer.com/html/products. html.

A third way to import and translate data is to use syntax (i.e., a computer program), which specifies the commands necessary to read the ASCII or other data set and translate it into a format usable by the statistical analysis package. This method has the advantages that the syntax may be shared among users, may be rerun if a file is lost or damaged, and may often be reused with minor modifications from year to year if a data set is released annually in a consistent format. Many of the federal data sets described in this book are supplied with syntax to convert the ASCII file to one or more proprietary formats, most often SPSS, SAS, and/or Stata. Another great advantage of using syntax is that it generally includes assignment statements for variable and value labels, which saves a lot of time and spares the analyst from having to enter these labels manually.

The process may be easier to explain if we consider an example. Data from the 2005 National Health Interview Survey is available for download in ASCII format from http://www.cdc.gov/nchs/about/major/nhis/nhis_2005_data_release.htm. The same web page contains links to SAS, SPSS, and Stata syntax that will convert the ASCII file to one of three proprietary formats. The necessary steps to make the data usable in one of those programs are as follows:

1. Download the ASCII file.
2. Download the relevant program.
3. Alter the program to match the local computing environment.
4. Run the program, creating a file in the chosen format that can then be used for further analysis.

The beginning of the ASCII file looks like this:

```
602005000002010038902005011122  2       12       10200022212108
1011011011012001010001010000200200200101200200200  0000
2002001021012002002002002001012002006091 200200200
```

The SAS, SPSS, and Stata programs all perform the same basic functions to convert this ASCII file to a specific format: the differences are due to details in the requirements of the proprietary program. For this reason, only one example is annotated here, the SPSS program. It should be easy to understand the other two programs by bearing in mind that they accomplish the same basic processes. In addition, because this program is quite lengthy (remember, a major reason to use the program is to avoid having to type all the variable names and labels), it is presented in excerpted form. Where lines have been omitted, the [**LINES OMITTED**] symbol appears. This program was downloaded from the previously cited website. My annotations are numbered in boldface and appear below the program.

```
*************************************************************(1)
* JUNE 20, 2006
*
* THIS IS AN EXAMPLE OF AN SPSS SCRIPT THAT CREATES
* A TEMPORARY SPSS FILE FROM THE
```

```
* 2005 NHIS PUBLIC USE familyxx.DAT ASCII FILE
*
* THIS IS STORED IN familyxx.SPS                          (2)
****************************************************************
FILE HANDLE TEMP                                          (3)
   /NAME='C:\NHIS2005\familyxx.dat'
   /RECFORM=VARIABLE
   /LRECL=176
DATA LIST FILE=TEMP FIXED RECORDS=1 TABLE /               (4)
   RECTYPE      1 -   2         SRVY_YR     3 -   6
   HHX          7 -  12 (A)     FMX        13 -  14 (A)
   WTFA_FAM    15 -  20
   FINT_Y_P    21 -  24         FINT_M_P   25 -  26
```

[LINES OMITTED]

```
   VARIABLE LABELS                                        (5)
   RECTYPE    "File type identifier"
   SRVY_YR    "Year of National Health Interview Survey"
   HHX        "HH identifier"
   FMX        "Family #"
   WTFA_FAM   "Weight - Final Annual"
   FINT_Y_P   "Date of Interview - Year"
```

[LINES OMITTED]

```
   VALUE LABELS                                           (6)
   RECTYPE
       10      "Household"
       20      "Person"
       30      "Sample Adult"
       31      "Sample Adult Cancer"
       40      "Sample Child"
       60      "Family"
       70      "Injury/Poisoning Episode"
       75      "Injury/Poisoning Verbatim"
/SRVY_YR
       2005    "2005"
/FINT_Y_P
       2005    "Year 2005"
       2006    "Year 2006"
"Not ascertained"
```

```
[LINES OMITTED]
FREQUENCIES GENERAL = RECTYPE.                          (7)
EXECUTE.                                                (8)
```

1. Lines beginning with an asterisk are comments, meaning that they do not execute but are there to give you information about the program and the files.

2. The suggested name for this syntax file is "familyxx.sps", and you will change the "xx" to correspond to the year; for instance, "family05.sps" for 2005 data. The extension ".sps" identifies an SPSS syntax file.

3. This FILE HANDLE command assigns the name TEMP to the physical storage location "C:\NHIS2005\familyxx.dat"; the location must be changed to match the actual storage location of the ASCII file on your computer, if necessary. The name TEMP is arbitrary and can be changed, but if it is changed here, it must then be changed throughout the program.

4. The DATA LIST FILE statement reads the ASCII file and assigns variable names to the contents of particular columns (because this is a fixed field file, as specified by the subcommand FIXED); for instance, the variable RECTYPE is read from columns 1 and 2.

5. The VARIABLE LABELS command associates longer descriptive phrases with the variable names assigned in the DATA FILE statement; for instance, the label for the variable SRVY_YR is "Year of National Health Interview Survey". These labels contain more information than the variable names and can be made to appear in some SPSS procedures instead of the variable name.

6. The VALUE LABELS command assigns descriptive labels to individual values of specific variables: for instance, for the variable RECTYPE, value "10" is labeled "Household", value 20 is labeled "Person", and value 30 is labeled "Sample Adult". These labels are more informative than the numeric codes stored in the data set and can be made to appear in some SPSS procedures instead of the codes. The section containing labels for each variable is demarcated with a slash (/), so "/ SRVY_YR" signals the beginning of the labels for the variable SRVY_YR.

7. The FREQUENCIES command will produce a frequency table for the variable RECTYPE; you can change this to produce a frequency table on any variable.

8. EXECUTE will cause the program to run; it is not necessary if the previous FREQUENCIES command is included in the file.

VERY IMPORTANT: As the comment at the beginning of the file states, this program creates a *temporary* SPSS file that will be lost when you shut down the SPSS program if you do not save it as a permanent SPSS data set with an exact location. This can be done through the menu system (select File>Save) or through syntax. SPSS data sets have the extension ".sav", so your permanent file should have a name such as "family05.sav". Although there are several ways to save SPSS files using syntax, one is to add the following commands to the end of the program. This would save the temporary SPSS file to the permanent location "C:\NHIS2005\SPSS data\family05.sav", assuming you are using a Windows computer and the folders "C:\NHIS2005\SPSS data\" already exists on your computer. The name of the data file in this case is "family05.sav".

```
FILE HANDLE family05
  /NAME='C:\NHIS2005\SPSS data\family05.sav'.
SAVE OUTFILE = family05.
EXECUTE.
```

Bibliography

Many of the data sets discussed in this volume are described and/or analyzed in one or more National Center for Health Statistics (NCHS) reports. Because of space limitations (there are literally hundreds of these reports), they are not included in this bibliography, but a complete list and links to downloadable texts of these reports are available from the NCHS website at http://www.cdc.gov/nchs/products/pubs/pubd/series/ser.htm.

Chapter 1. An Introduction to Secondary Data Analysis

Black N. 2003. Secondary use of personal data for health and health services research: Why identifiable data are essential. *Journal of Health Services Research & Policy* 8(Suppl 1):36–40.

Bulmer MIA, Sturgis PJ, Allum N. 2006. *The secondary analysis of survey data.* Thousand Oaks, CA: Sage.

Ciol MA, Hoffman JM, Dudgeon BJ, Shumway-Cook A, Yorkston KM, Chan L. 2006. Understanding the use of weights in the analysis of data from multistage surveys. *Archives of Physical Medicine and Rehabilitation* 87(2):299–303.

de Vaus D. 2002. *Social surveys.* Thousand Oaks, CA: Sage.

Elder GH, Pavalko EK, Clipp EC. 1993. *Working with archival data: Studying lives.* Thousand Oaks, CA: Sage.

Heaton J. 2004. *Reworking qualitative data.* Thousand Oaks, CA: Sage.

Hinds P, Vogel R, Clarke-Steffen L. 1997. The possibilities and pitfalls of doing a secondary analysis of a qualitative data set. *Qualitative Health Research* 7(3):408–424.

Huston P, Naylor CD. 1996. Health services research: Reporting on studies using secondary data. *Canadian Medical Association Journal* 155(12):1697–1702.

James J, Sorensen A. 2000. Archiving longitudinal data for future research: Why qualitative data add to a study's usefulness. *Forum: Qualitative Social Research* 1(3). Available online at: http://qualitative-research.net/fqs/fqs-eng.htm. Accessed July 6, 2006.

Jiang Y, Alastair JS, Wild CJ. 2006. Secondary analysis of case-control data. *Statistics in Medicine* 25:1323–1339.

Lee AJ, McMurchy L, Scott AJ. 1997. Re-using data from case-control studies. *Statistics in Medicine* 16:1377–1389.

Lowrance WW. 2003. Learning from experience: Privacy and the secondary use of data in health research. *Journal of Biolaw and Business* 6(4):30–60.

Kiekolt KJ, Nathan LE. 1985. *Secondary analysis of survey data.* Thousand Oaks, CA: Sage.

Pearl J. 2000. *Causality.* New York: Cambridge University Press.

Phillips CV, Goodman KJ. 2006. Causal criteria and counterfactuals: Nothing more (or less) than scientific common sense. *Emerging Themes in Epidemiology* 3:5. Available online at: http://www.ete-online.com/content/3/1/5. Accessed September 20, 2006.

Rothman KJ, Greenland S. 1998. *Modern epidemiology.* 2nd ed. Philadelphia: Lippincott.

Sieber JE, ed. 1991. *Sharing social science data: Advantages and challenges.* Thousand Oaks, CA: Sage.

Stewart E, Kamins MA. 1992. *Secondary research: Information sources and methods.* 2nd ed. Thousand Oaks, CA: Sage.

Tomlinson-Keasey CA. 1993. Opportunities and challenges posed by archival data sets. In: Funder DC, Parke RD, Tomlinson-Keasey CA, Widaman L, eds. *Studying lives through time: Personality and development.* Washington, DC: American Psychological Association, pp. 65–92.

Yeager KR, Roberts AR. 2006. Mental illness, substance dependence, and suicidality: Secondary data analysis. In: Roberts AR, Yeager KR, eds. *Foundations of evidence-based social work practice.* New York: Oxford, pp. 314–322.

Chapter 2. Health Services Utilization Data

Bartlett DL, Ezzati-Rice TM, Stokley S, Zhao Z. 2001. Comparison of NIS and NHIS/NIPRCS vaccination coverage estimates. *American Journal of Preventive Medicine* 20(4 Suppl):25–27.

Bradley CJ, Neumark D, Oberst K, Luo Z, Brennan S, Schenk M. 2005. Combining registry, primary, and secondary data sources to identify the impact of cancer on labor market outcomes. *Medical Decision Making* 25(5):534–547.

Gilchrist VJ, Stange KC, Flocke SA, McCord G, Bourguet CC. 2004. A comparison of the National Ambulatory Medical Care Survey (NAMCS) measurement approach with direct observation of outpatient visits. *Medical Care* 42(3):276–280.

Hing E, Gousen S, Shimizu I, Burt C. 2003. Guide to using masked design variables to estimate standard errors in public use files of the National Ambulatory Medical Care Survey and the National Hospital Ambulatory Medical Care Survey. *Inquiry* 40(4):401–415.

Luo YH, Zack M. 2005. Computations of confidence intervals for estimates in the United States National Hospital Discharge Survey, 1979–2000. *Preventing Chronic Disease* 2(3):A06. Epub 2005 Jun 15.

Merrill RM, Dearden KA. 2004. How representative are the surveillance, epidemiology, and end results (SEER) program cancer data of the United States? *Cancer Causes & Control* 15(10):1027–1034.

Smith PJ, Battaglia MP, Huggins VJ, Hoaglin DC, Roden A, Khare M, Ezzati-Rice TA, Wright RA. 2001. Overview of the sampling design and statistical methods used in the National Immunization Survey. *American Journal of Preventive Medicine* 20(4 Suppl):17–24.

Steiner C, Elixhauser A, Schnaier J. 2002. The Healthcare Cost and Utilization Project: An overview. *Effective Clinical Practice* 5(3):143–151.

Zell ER, Ezzati-Rice TM, Battaglia MP, Wright RA. 2000. National Immunization Survey: The methodology of a vaccination surveillance system. *Public Health Reports* 115(1):65–77.

Chapter 3. Health Behaviors and Risk Factors Data

Andresen EM, Catlin TK, Wyrwich KW, Jackson-Thompson J. 2003. Re-test reliability of surveillance questions on health related quality of life. *Journal of Epidemiology and Community Health* 57(5):339–343.

Bowlin SJ, Morril BD, Nafziger AN, Jenkins PL, Lewis C, Pearson TA. 1993. Validity of cardiovascular disease risk factors assessed by telephone survey: The Behavioral Risk Factor Survey. *Journal of Clinical Epidemiology* 46(6):561–571.

Brener ND, Kann L, Kinchen SA, Grunbaum JA, Whalen L, Eaton D, Hawkins J, Ross JG. 2004. Methodology of the Youth Risk Behavior Surveillance System. *MMWR Recommendations and Reports* 53(RR-12):1–13.

Gentry EM, Kalsbeek WD, Hogelin GC, Jones JT, Gaines KL, Forman MR, Marks JS, Trowbridge FL. 1985. The Behavioral Risk Factor Surveys: II. Design, methods, and estimates from combined state data. *American Journal of Preventive Medicine* 1(6):9–14.

Johnston LD, O'Malley PM. 1997. The recanting of earlier reported drug use by young adults. *NIDA Research Monograph* 167:59–80.

O'Malley PM, Bachman JG, Johnston LD. 1983. Reliability and consistency in self-reports of drug use. *International Journal of the Addictions* 18(6):805–824.

Nelson DE, Holtzman D, Bolen J, Stanwyck CA, Mack KA. 2001. Reliability and validity of measures from the Behavioral Risk Factor Surveillance System (BRFSS). *Social and Preventive Medicine* 46(Suppl 1):S3–S42.

Remington PL, Smith MY, Williamson DF, Anda RF, Gentry EM, Hogelin GC. 1988. Design, characteristics, and usefulness of state-based behavioral risk factor surveillance 1981–1987. *Public Health Reports* 103(4):366–375.

Chapter 4. Data on Multiple Health Topics

Fronstin P. 2000. Counting the uninsured: A comparison of national surveys. *Employee Benefit Research Institute Issue Brief* 225:1–19.

Himes JH, Faricy A. 2001. Validity and reliability of self-reported stature and weight of US adolescents. *American Journal of Human Biology* 13(2):255–260.

James MK, Miller ME, Anderson RT, Worley AS, Longino CF Jr. 1997. Benefits of linkage to the National Death Index in the Longitudinal Study of Aging. *Journal of Aging and Health* 9(3):298–315.

Korenman S, Goldman N, Fu H. 1997. Misclassification bias in estimates of bereavement effects. *American Journal of Epidemiology* 145(11):995–1002.

Kuczmarski MF, Kuczmarski RJ, Najjar M. 2001. Effects of age on validity of self-reported height, weight, and body mass index: Findings from the Third National Health and Nutrition Examination Survey, 1988–1994. *Journal of the American Dietetic Association* 101(1):28–34.

Vargas CM, Burt VL, Gillum RF, Pamuk ER. 1997. Validity of self-reported hypertension in the National Health and Nutrition Examination Survey III, 1988–1991. *Preventive Medicine* 26(5 Pt 1):678–685.

Yabroff KR, Gordis L. 2003. Assessment of a national health interview survey-based method of measuring community socioeconomic status. *Annals of Epidemiology* 13(10):721–726.

Chapter 5. Fertility and Mortality Data

Adams M. 2001. Validity of birth certificate data for the outcome of the previous pregnancy, Georgia, 1980–1995. *American Journal of Epidemiology* 154(10):883–888.

Baumeister L, Marchi K, Pearl M, Williams R, Braveman P. 2000. The validity of information on "race" and "Hispanic ethnicity" in California birth certificate data. *Health Services Research* 35(4):869–883.

Campbell AA, Mosher WD. 2000. A history of the measurement of unintended pregnancies and births. *Maternal and Child Health Journal* 4(3):163–169.

Cowper DC, Kubal JD, Maynard C, Hynes DM. 2002. A primer and comparative review of major US mortality databases. *Annals of Epidemiology* 12(7):462–468.

DiGiuseppe DL, Aron DC, Ranbom L, Harper DL, Rosenthal GE. 2002. Reliability of birth certificate data: A multi-hospital comparison to medical records information. *Maternal and Child Health Journal* 6(3):169–179.

Johansson LA, Westerling R, Rosenberg HM. 2006. Methodology of studies evaluating death certificate accuracy were flawed. *Journal of Clinical Epidemiology* 59(2):125–131.

Kaufmann RB, Morris L, Spitz AM. 1997. Comparison of two question sequences for assessing pregnancy intentions. *American Journal of Epidemiology* 145(9):810–816.

Klerman LV. 2000. The intendedness of pregnancy: A concept in transition. *Maternal and Child Health Journal* 4(3):155–162.

Lydon-Rochelle MT, Cardenas V, Nelson JL, Tomashek KM, Mueller BA, Easterling TR. 2005. Validity of maternal and perinatal risk factors reported on fetal death certificates. *American Journal of Public Health* 95(11):1948–1951.

Lydon-Rochelle MT, Holt VL, Nelson JC, Cardenas V, Gardella C, Easterling TR, Callaghan WM. 2005. Accuracy of reporting maternal in-hospital diagnoses and intrapartum procedures in Washington State linked birth records. *Paediatric and Perinatal Epidemiology* 19(6):460–471.

Martin JA, Hoyert DL. 2002. The national fetal death file. *Seminars in Perinatology* 26(1):3–11.

Mosher WD. 1998. Design and operation of the 1995 National Survey of Family Growth. *Family Planning Perspectives* 30(1):43–46.

Northam S, Knapp TR. 2006. The reliability and validity of birth certificates. *Journal of Obstetric, Gynecologic and Neonatal Nursing* 35(1):3–12.

Rothwell CJ. 2004. Reengineering vital registration and statistics systems for the United States. *Preventing Chronic Disease* 1(4):A03. Epub 2004 Sep 15.

Shulman HB, Gilbert BC, Msphbrenda CG, Lansky A. 2006. The Pregnancy Risk Assessment Monitoring System (PRAMS): Current methods and evaluation of 2001 response rates. *Public Health Reports* 121(1):74–83.

Chapter 6. Medicare and Medicaid Data

Cooper GS, Yuan Z, Stange KC, Amini SB, Dennis LK, Rimm AA. 1999. The utility of Medicare claims data for measuring cancer stage. *Medical Care* 37(7):706–711.

Chattopadhyay A, Bindman AB. 2005. Accuracy of Medicaid payer coding in hospital patient discharge data: Implications for Medicaid policy evaluation. *Medical Care* 43(6):586–591.

Doctor JN, Chan L, MacLehose RF, Patrick DL. 2000. Weighted health status in the Medicare population: Development of the Weighted Health Index for the Medicare Current Beneficiary Survey (WHIM-CBS). *Journal of Outcome Measurement* 4(4):721–739.

Fisher ES, Baron JA, Malenka DJ, Barrett J, Bubolz TA. 1990. Overcoming potential pitfalls in the use of Medicare data for epidemiologic research. *American Journal of Public Health* 80(12):1487–1490.

Gyllstrom ME, Jensen JL, Vaughan JN, Castellano SE, Oswald JW. 2002. Linking birth certificates with Medicaid data to enhance population health assessment: Methodological issues addressed. *Journal of Public Health Management and Practice* 8(4):38–44.

Hoffman ED, Klees BS, Curtis CA. 2002. Overview of the Medicare and Medicaid programs. *Health Care Financing Review Statistical Supplement* 1–348.

Jones N III, Jones SL, Miller NA. 2004. The Medicare Health Outcomes Survey program: Overview, context, and near-term prospects. *Health and Quality of Life Outcomes* 2:33. Available online at: http://www.hqlo.com/content/2/1/33. Accessed July 6, 2006.

Koroukian SM, Cooper GS, Alfred, Rimm AA. 2002. Ability of Medicaid claims data to identify incident cases of breast cancer in the Ohio Medicaid population. *Health Services Research* 38(3):947–960.

Morgan RO, Wei II, Virnig BA. 2004. Improving identification of Hispanic males in Medicare: Use of surname matching. *Medical Care* 42(8):810–816.

Saydah SH, Geiss LS, Tierney E, Benjamin SM, Engelgau M, Brancati F. 2004. Review of the performance of methods to identify diabetes cases among vital statistics, administrative, and survey data. *Annals of Epidemiology* 14(7):507–516.

Wang PS, Walker A, Tsuang M, Orav EJ, Levin R, Avorn J. 2000. Strategies for improving comorbidity measures based on Medicare and Medicaid claims data. *Journal of Clinical Epidemiology* 53(6):571–578.

Weiner M, Stump TE, Callahan CM, Lewis JN, McDonald CJ. 2003. A practical method of linking data from Medicare claims and a comprehensive electronic medical records system. *International Journal of Medical Informatics* 71(1):57–69.

Wunsch H, Harrison DA, Rowan K. 2005. Health services research in critical care using administrative data. *Journal of Critical Care* 20(3):264–269.

Zhan C, Miller MR. 2003. Administrative data based patient safety research: A critical review. *Quality and Safety in Health Care* 12(Suppl 2): 58–63.

Chapter 7. Other Sources of Data

Barrett RE. 1994. *Using the 1990 U.S. Census for Research.* Thousand Oaks, CA: Sage.

Best AE. 1999. Secondary data bases and their use in outcomes research: A review of the Area Resource File and the Healthcare Cost and Utilization Project. *Journal of Medical Systems* 23(3):175–181.

Davis J. 1991. *The NORC General Social Survey: A user's guide.* Thousand Oaks, CA: Sage.

A Guide to the Data Resources of the Henry A. Murray Research Center of Radcliffe College, A Center for the Study of Lives. 1996. Cambridge, MA: Radcliffe Institutes for Advanced Study.

Mays VM, Ponce NA, Washington DL, Cochran SD. 2003. Classification of race and ethnicity: Implications for public health. *Annual Review of Public Health* 24:83–110.

Van der Heijden PJM, van Puijenbroek EP, van Buuren S, van der Hofstede JW. 2002. On the assessment of adverse drug reactions from spontaneous reporting systems: The influence of under-reporting on odds ratios. *Statistics in Medicine* 21:2027–2044.

Young CH, Savola KL, Phelps E. 1991. *Inventory of longitudinal studies in the social sciences.* Thousand Oaks, CA: Sage.

Index